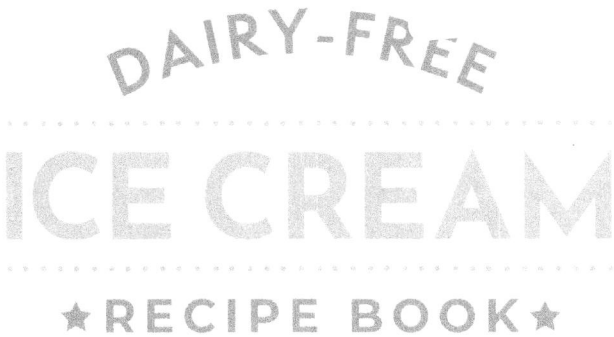

101 Delicious Frozen Desserts to Make At Home!

EDITION 3

By Lisa Brian

healthy happy Foodie

HHF Press
San Francisco

COPYRIGHT © 2022 Healthy Happy Foodie Press (HHF Press)

First published 2022

All rights reserved. No part of this book may be reproduced in any form or by any electronic or mechanical means, including information storage and retrieval systems, without permission in writing from the publisher, except by reviewers, who may quote brief passages in a review.

Editor: HHF Press

Art Direction: HHF Press

Illustrations: HHF Press

All photographs in this book © HHF Press or © Depositphotos.com

Published in the United States of America by HHF Press

www.HHFPress.com

Disclaimer:

Although the publisher and authors of this book are practically obsessed with modern cooking techniques, neither the publisher nor the authors represent or are affiliated with any of the brands mentioned in this text.

All content herein represents the authors' own experiences and opinions, and do not represent medical or health advice. The responsibility for the consequences of your actions, including your use or misuse of any suggestion or procedure described in this book lies not with the authors, publisher or distributors of this book. We recommend using common sense and consulting with a licensed health professional before changing your diet or exercise. The authors or the publisher do not assume any liability for the use of or inability to use any or all of the information contained in this book, nor do the authors or publisher accept responsibility for any type of loss or damage that may be experienced by the user as the result of activities occurring from the use of any information in this book. Use the information responsibly and at your own risk.

The authors and publisher reserve the right to make changes he or she deems required to future versions of the publication to maintain accuracy.

CONTENTS

WHY YOU NEED THIS BOOK	1
WHY USE A FROZEN TREAT MAKER?	5
HEALTH BENEFITS OF FRUIT BASED FROZEN DESSERTS	8
HOW TO USE YOUR FROZEN TREAT MAKER	12
PRO TIPS TO MAKE PERFECT SOFT-SERVE DESSERT	15
HOW TO STORE YOUR SOFT-SERVE DESSERTS	18
RECIPES	20
Marmalade Ice Cream	22
Bourbon Ice Cream	23
Mojito Sorbet	24
Lime-Basil Sorbet	25
Zucchini-Lemon Sorbet	26
Raspberry-Campari Sorbet	27
Pink Grapefruit Sorbet	28
Blueberry Cheesecake Ice Cream	29
Almond Nougat Mousse Ice Cream	30
Apple Sorbet	32
Mango Tango	33
Pumpkin Pie Ice Cream	34
Pineapple Sorbet	35
Raspberry and Redcurrant Sorbet	36
Coconut Caramel Ice Cream	38
Chocolate-Coffee Ice Cream	40
Brownie Batter No-Churn Ice Cream	41
Bananas with Toasted Coconut, Almonds, & Dark Chocolate	42
Red Plum Sorbet	43
Mint Chocolate Chip Ice Cream	45
Caramelized Pecan Banana "Ice Cream" with Chocolate Hazelnut	46
Dark Choco-Peanut Butter Ice Cream	2
Iced Coffee with Banana Ice Cream and Caramel Sauce	3
Berry Ice Cream with Banana Meringue	4
Peanut Butter Pretzel Ice Cream	5
Spiced Apple Cider Sorbet	6
Chocolate Ice Cream	8
Lavender Coconut Ice Cream	9
Sugar-free Coconut Vanilla Ice Cream	10
Choco-Chunk Banana Ice Cream with Choco-Fudge Ripple	11

Pumpkin Cookie Ice Cream	13
Chocolate Peanut Butter Banana Ice Cream	14
Peanut Butter Frozen Banana	15
Strawberry Banana Ice Cream	17
Blueberry-Basil-Banana Soft-Serve	18
Pistachio Frozen Treat	19
Date, Rum, & Pecan Ice Cream	20
Vanilla Avocado Banana Ice Cream	21
Guinness-Milk Chocolate Ice Cream	22
Sweet Corn Ice Cream	23
Almond-Banana Ice Cream	24
S'mores Ice Cream Sandwiches	25
Peach Ice Cream	26
Concord Grape Sorbet	27
Salted Caramel Ice Cream	28
Coconut-Rum Ice Cream	29
Huckleberry Ice Cream	30
Peanut Butter Ice Cream	31
Kaffir Lime Gelato	32
PawPaw Ice Cream	33
Banana Ice Cream with Walnut Chip	34
Banana-Raisin Froyo	35
Blueberry Banana Ice Cream	36
Banana Ice Cream with Cashew and Almond	37
Neapolitan Banana Ice Cream	38
Pumpkin Soft-Serve with Candied Ginger and Dark Chocolate	39
Almond Torte Mascarpone Ice Cream	40
Rum and Raisin Ice Cream	41
Homemade Coco-Mango Sorbet	42
Citrus-Mint Sorbet	43
Blueberry Frozen Soy Yogurt	44
Cherry-Coconut Ice Cream Sandwiches	45
Malted Milk Ice Cream Bonbons	46
Cookie Dough Ice Cream	47
Lemon Buttermilk Pie Ice Cream	48
Vegan Coconut Raspberry Ice Cream	49
Coconut Cake Frosting Ice Cream	50
Lemon-Aid Sorbet	51
Maple Bacon Ice Cream	52
Chiquita Banana Ice Cream	53
Passion Fruit Ice Cream	54
Non-Dairy Peach Ice Cream	55
Rosé Sherbet	56

Banana Nutella Soft-Serve	57
Fried Ice Cream	58
Root Beer Barrel Ice Cream	59
Chocolate Decadence Ice Cream	60
Oat & Dulce de Leche Sorbet	61
Orange Ice Cream with Dark Chocolate Chip	62
Peach Ice Cream	63
Tahini and Lemon Curd Ice Cream	64
Chocolate Malted Whopper Ice Cream	65
Banana Sorbet with Rose and Pistachio	66
Cinnamon Cream Cheese Ice Cream	67
Stracciatella Ice Cream	68
Berry Ice Cream with Goat Cheese	69
Red Velvet Ice Cream	70
Macaroon Ice Cream Torte	71
Lemongrass Ginger Coconut Ice Cream	72
Watermelon Ice Cream	73
Rhubarb Ice Cream	74
Peanut Butter and Jelly Ice Cream	75
Amaretto-Coffee Ice Cream	76
Banana-Coconut Ice Cream	77
Lemon Drop Sorbet	78
Chocolate Coconut Ice Cream Sandwiches	79
Chocolate Hazelnut Ice Cream	80
Sweet Corn Ice Cream	81
Cookies and Ice Cream	82
Fruity Frozen Yogurt	83
BONUS	**84**

CHAPTER 1
Why You Need This Book

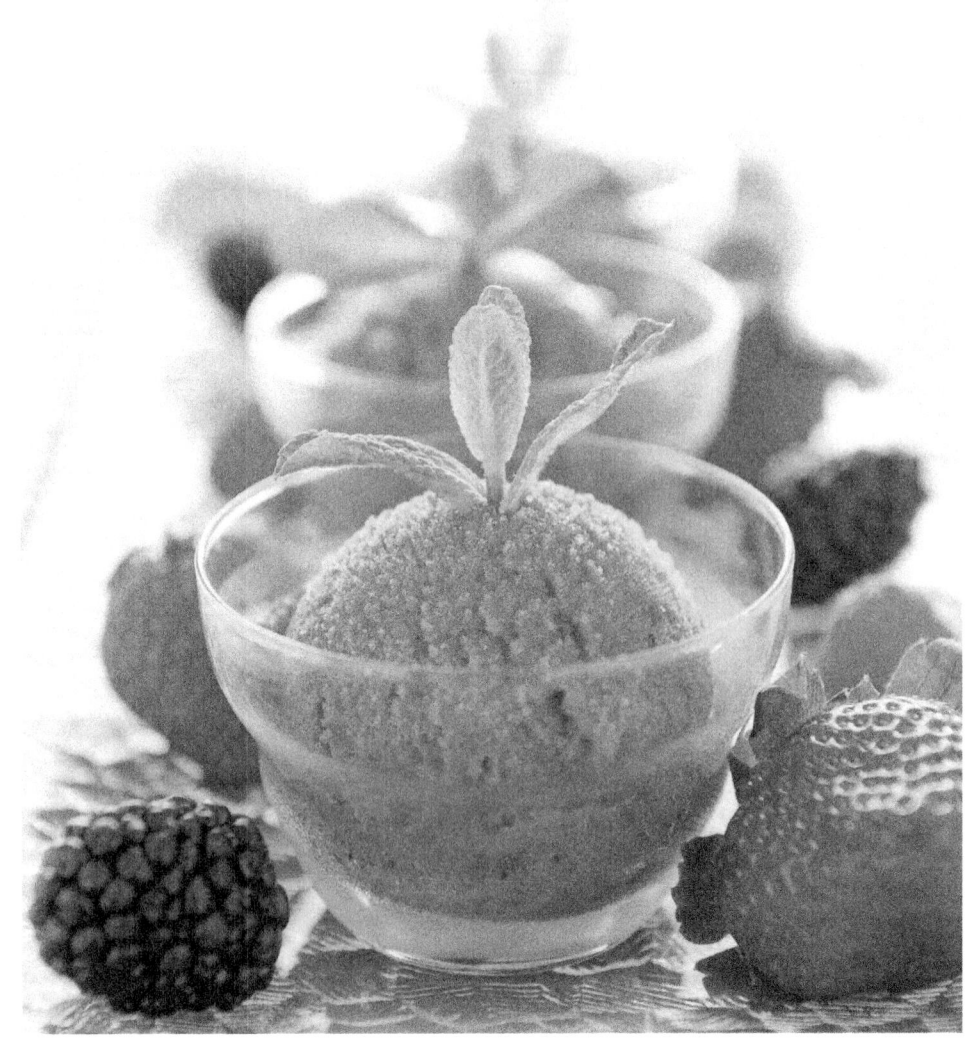

This Book Will Teach You Everything You Need to Know About Getting the Most Out of Your Frozen Treat Maker

While your frozen treat maker surely comes with a guide, it doesn't come with pro tips, 101 delicious recipes, the best fruit to use, or how to prep fruit for the best soft-serve experience using your frozen treat maker If you're looking for more ways to get the most out of your frozen treat making experience, this book has everything you need and more when it comes to enhancing your healthy lifestyle.

A Wealth of Valuable Information

Not only will you learn what to do with your frozen treat maker the moment you open the box, you'll learn the benefits of the delicious recipes too! You'll get detailed information for your frozen treat maker, plus loads of pro tips to make the perfect soft-serve right at home. The wealth of information on health benefits alone make this book worth reading.

101 New Delicious, Scrumptious Recipes to Try Out

While your frozen treat maker probably comes with a few recipes, we've got 101 delicious, scrumptious and decadent ways for you to make the best healthy soft-serve right in your own home. Think: ice cream that is super healthy with no added sugars, diabetic friendly recipes, and recipes for those days when you want to splurge and still stay on your diet.

These quick and easy recipes also come with pro tips on how to make the most out of each bowl and will have you serving up healthy soft-serve to the whole family in no time.

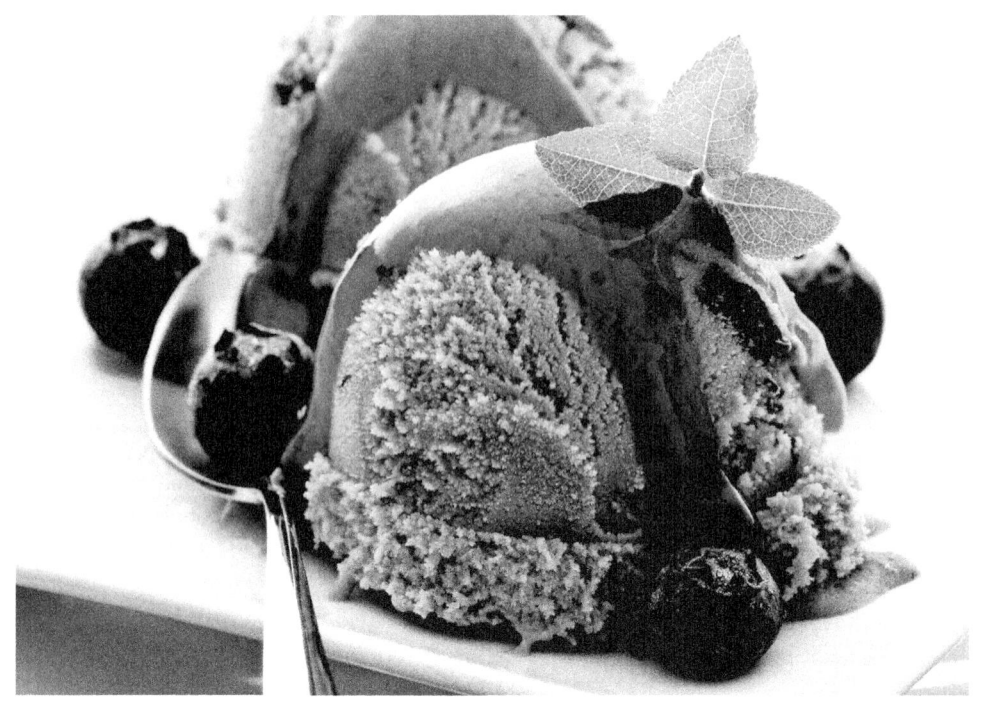

A Whole New World of Healthy Desserts

Soft-serve ice cream is what you will think of, from now on, when someone says "healthy dessert." Once you try fruit based soft-serve, you'll want to try every single extraordinary recipe in this book. With the base of the soft serve being bananas, even if you add your own decadent ingredients, this is a very healthy treat. Not only is it compatible with most diets and natural lifestyles, you'll get an extra serving of amazing super-foods for a delicious healthy boost to your daily diet.

Lose Weight Through Clean Eating!

Dieting is super-fun when you use your frozen treat maker. Now, you can join any of the new clean-living revolutions and not pack on any extra weight! Fruit based soft-serve is so diet-friendly that you can enjoy it no matter what sort of healthy lifestyle you lead. From gluten-free to paleo, clean and raw eating, there are just as many reasons to start making fruit-based soft-serve as there are recipes in this book.

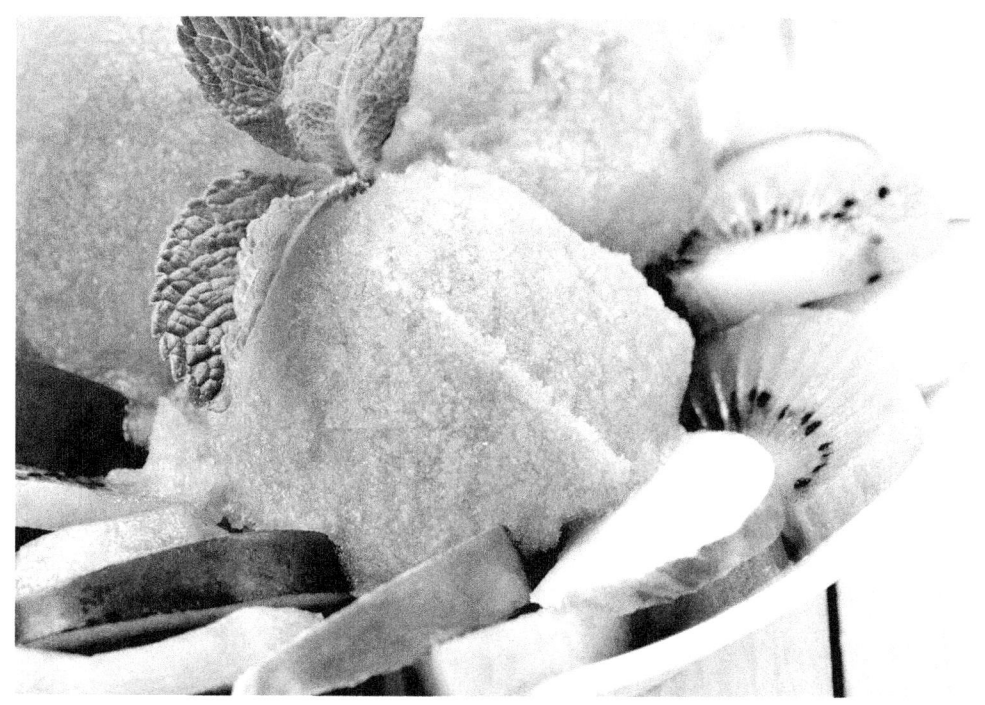

This Book is For SO MUCH MORE Than Bananas!

The amazing thing about your frozen treat maker is that it is for so much more than bananas. You can make whatever scrumptious, decadent, dreamy frozen treats your healthy heart desires with this book. Think: Brown Sugar Bourbon Ice Cream, Mojito Sorbet, Vegan Coconut Raspberry Ice Cream, Guinness Milk Chocolate Ice Cream, Salted Caramel—even Neapolitan Ice Cream. The possibilities are endless with this amazing book and its 101 recipes.

CHAPTER 2
Why Use a Frozen Treat Maker?

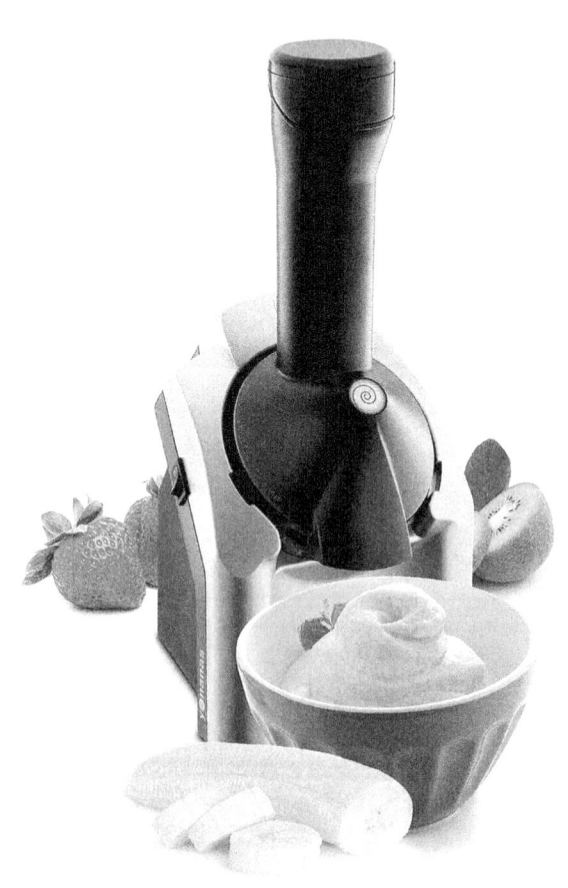

The Revolutionary Way to Enjoy Soft-Serve Right at Home

With your frozen treat maker you will make super-trendy, rich soft-serve right at home without the typical cost of such luxury. You can also top your soft-serve treats with healthier options, and decadent ones when you really have a hankering to fulfill your sweet tooth. Creating soft-serve in your own kitchen with your frozen treat maker also helps you choose healthier options and abstain from refined sugars. The best part about your frozen treat maker is that you decide what goes in it, and our 101 recipes can help you choose something blissfully perfect for your healthy lifestyle.

Super Diet-Friendly for a Plethora of Lifestyles

Think: lactose intolerant, vegan, gluten-free, paleo, raw, and clean eating. These treats are made from fruit, so they're 100% dairy free. You select the additives, so it's easier to stick to your own healthy eating plan. If you're a dieter who counts points, fruit based soft-serve is also a zero-points dessert. Plus, there are also a lot of great supplements you can use to modify recipes in order to make them more low-carb friendly or vegan. You'll find all those pro tips and tricks right here!

No Preservatives, GMOs, or Additives

With preservatives, GMOs and additives becoming some of the most avoided ingredients in food these days, fruit-based treats are the way to go! Traditional supermarket sorbet and ice cream often have a lot of ingredients that don't fit with your healthy lifestyle. Some are even made with gelatins not suitable for vegan or vegetarian lifestyles. Fruit based soft-serve desserts are made with 100% fresh fruit, so you can go totally organic, fresh and additive-free if you desire—with little to no effort. It's so easy, even kids love making soft-serve with your frozen treat maker.

Supports Weight Loss Lifestyles

One of the main ingredients in ruining your diet is sugar. Frozen treats are nearly impossible to find without some sort of added sugar or sugar substitute. Plus, they can be made with heavy cream making them high in fat content. Your frozen treat maker is the ultimate way to enjoy frozen treats without worrying about your weight, because the only sugar you get is from natural, freshly frozen fruit.

Super Easy to Use, Clean, and Maintain

Your frozen treat maker is easy to assemble, clean and maintain because it doesn't require a bunch of parts. There are some tips and tricks to go along with the easy cleaning that will help you, not only get the most out of the machine and your fruit, it will also help you maintain the machine for endless soft-serve making.

The Healthy Alternative to Ice Cream

Your frozen treat maker doesn't use any cream or milk-based products or added sugar unless you add them yourself. This fruit-based ice cream alternative is more of a sorbet than anything, but you'll never know the difference once you get into the 101 decadent recipes included. With all-natural ingredients and no additives, plus natural sugar and fiber from raw, frozen fruit, your frozen treat maker lets you produce delicious and healthy ice cream.

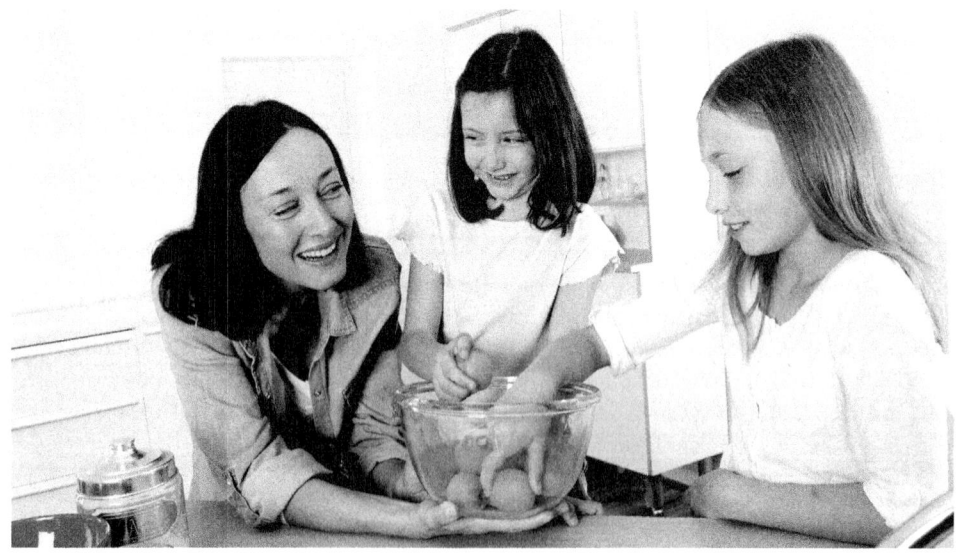

Your Frozen Treat Maker is Kid Friendly

Kids love playing in the kitchen or helping out to create their own foods.

Creating kid friendly activities in the kitchen is a breeze with your frozen treat maker. It's so easy to use, you'll just need to guide children until they get the hang of it. It's also a great way to teach children about clean and healthy eating, making your frozen treat maker perfect for kid friendly fun.

CHAPTER 3
Health Benefits of Fruit Based Frozen Desserts

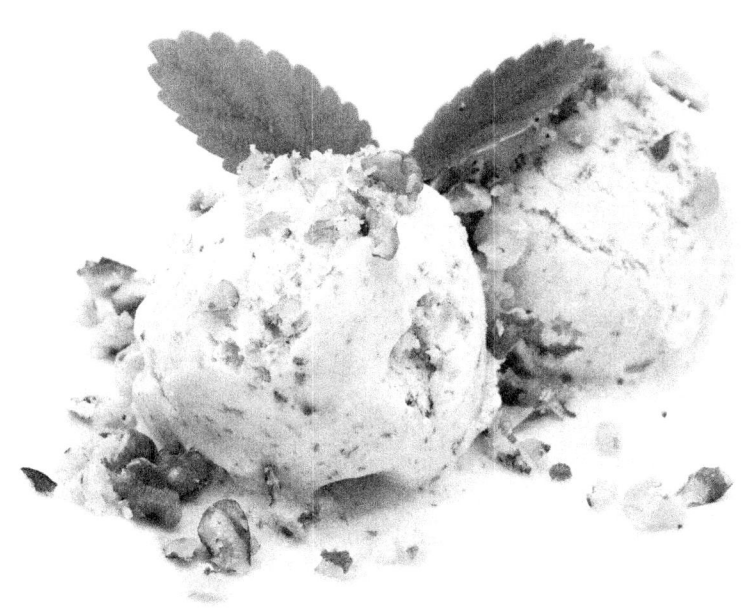

Packed With Loads of Antioxidants

You might know what antioxidants are, but do you know how awesome they are for your body? Fruit-based desserts are loaded with healthy antioxidants that come from fresh, frozen fruit. Antioxidants are proven to promote brain health, prevent dementia, increase blood flow to the brain, increase bone mass, help nurture your nervous system, improve learning and motor skills, protect the brain from damage-causing free radicals—and so much more! Antioxidants help your body naturally fight off disease and ageing for a super-healthy lifestyle.

A Great Way to Go on a Delicious Detox Diet

When our bodies consume a large amount of processed, packaged or canned foods we are adding a lot of unnecessary ingredients to our diet.

Consuming high amounts of sodium, complex carbohydrates and dairy found in processed and packaged foods can cause weight gain, as well as health problems like high cholesterol, high triglycerides, and high blood pressure—all symptoms of heart disease and diabetes. Not to mention the fact that your body doesn't break down dry food as well as it does fruit. Fruit based desserts can help you flush out your colon, liver and kidneys for a natural, delicious way to detox.

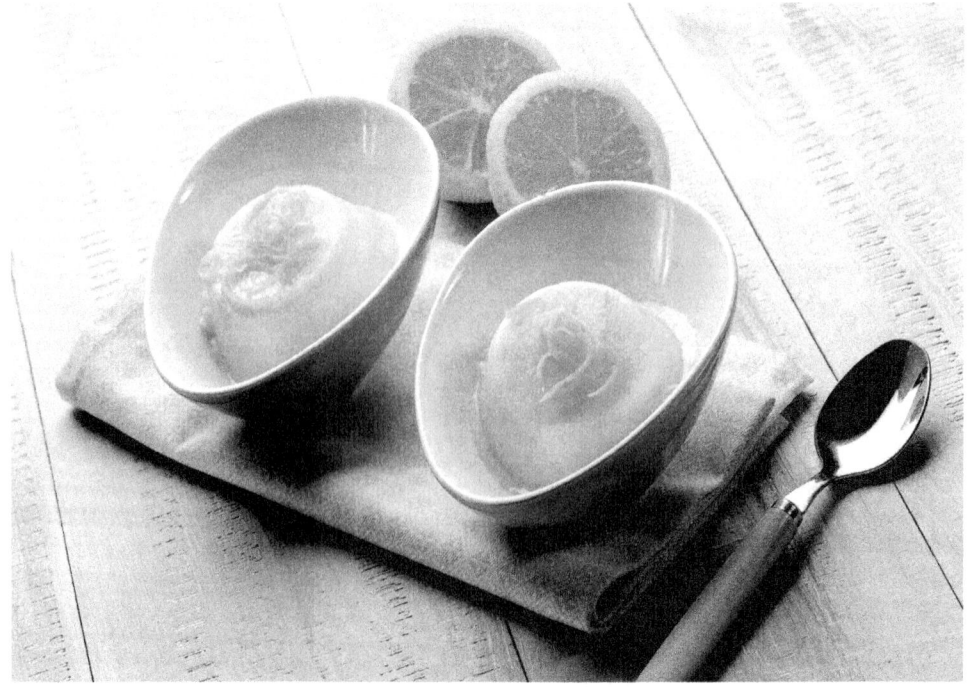

Helps Aid in Anti-Aging for Healthy, Glowing Skin

Have you ever thought of anti-aging from the inside out? Free radicals are introduced into our diet and cause our skin to age—it's that simple. Your frozen treat maker creates all natural, fruit based soft-serve is just the thing the dermatologist ordered. All those amazing antioxidants packed in your fruit based soft-serve not only give you a healthy mind, they can help aide in cellular skin repair for a healthier, all over glow.

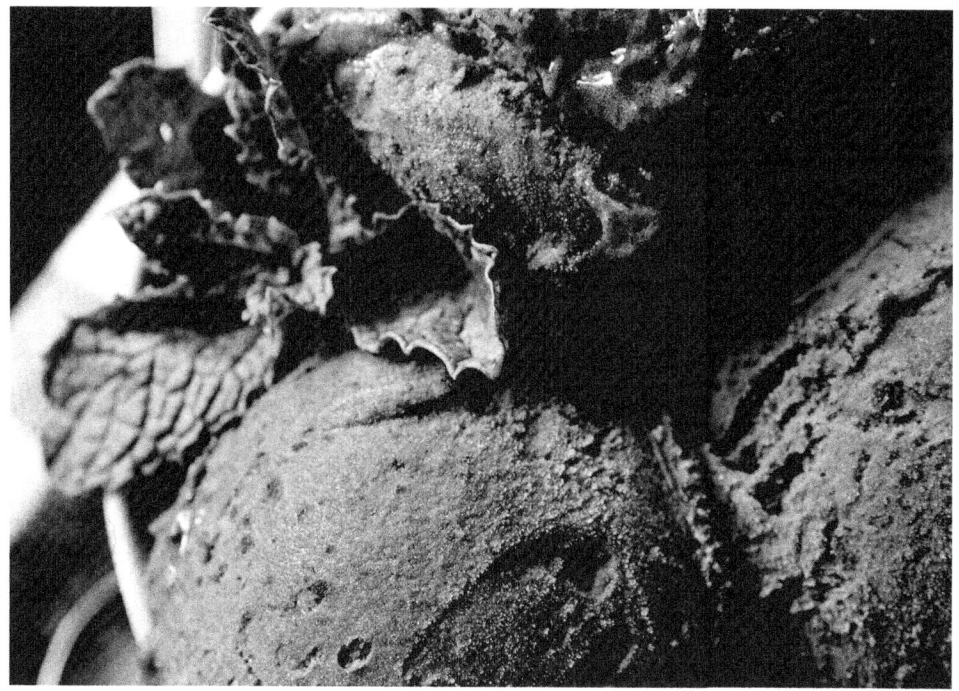

Packed with Vitamins, Minerals, and Fiber to Keep Your Body Healthy

Toss your daily vitamin and substitute delicious fruit based soft-serve instead! Combined with a healthy diet, fruit based soft-serve can help provide you with your daily dose of vitamins. The 101 recipes below feature fruits and ingredients that contain: Vitamin A; Vitamin B1, B2, B3, B6, B9 (folic acid); Vitamin C, E, and K. All fruit soft-serve is also packed with loads of minerals and fiber that can help aid in digestion, as well as absorption of healthy vitamins.

Can Fight Free Radicals that Cause Infections, Cancer, and Aging

Free radicals break down the cells in our body over time in a chain reaction, which causes your body to age. Essentially as you age your body becomes susceptible to infections, cancer and physical aging. How do you fight all that? With a healthy diet packed with fruits. One of the best ways to get your daily serving of scrumptious fruit is with a heavenly bowl of fruit based soft-serve. You'll think you're eating ice cream and forget how absolutely healthy it is and think more about what decadent recipe you want to try next!

Cool Down Your Body and Keep Hydrated

Fruit based soft-serve is the healthy way to cool down your body temperature during the hotter months or on scorching record temperature days. A great way to enjoy soft-serve in the heat is to check out the recipes that will keep you hydrated and cool on those super-hot summer days. Water-based fruits like watermelon, cantaloupe and oranges are great for hydration.

Increased Energy to Help You Take on the Day

Of course, fruit based soft-serve doesn't just hydrate. Some of the recipes are specifically designed to increase energy to help you take on the day. With all the superfoods you'll be consuming your increased energy will have you wanting to work it off in the gym, take a yoga class or join a fun workout class—getting you geared toward weight loss and a healthy lifestyle one delicious bowl of soft-serve ice cream after another.

CHAPTER 4
How to Use Your Frozen Treat Maker

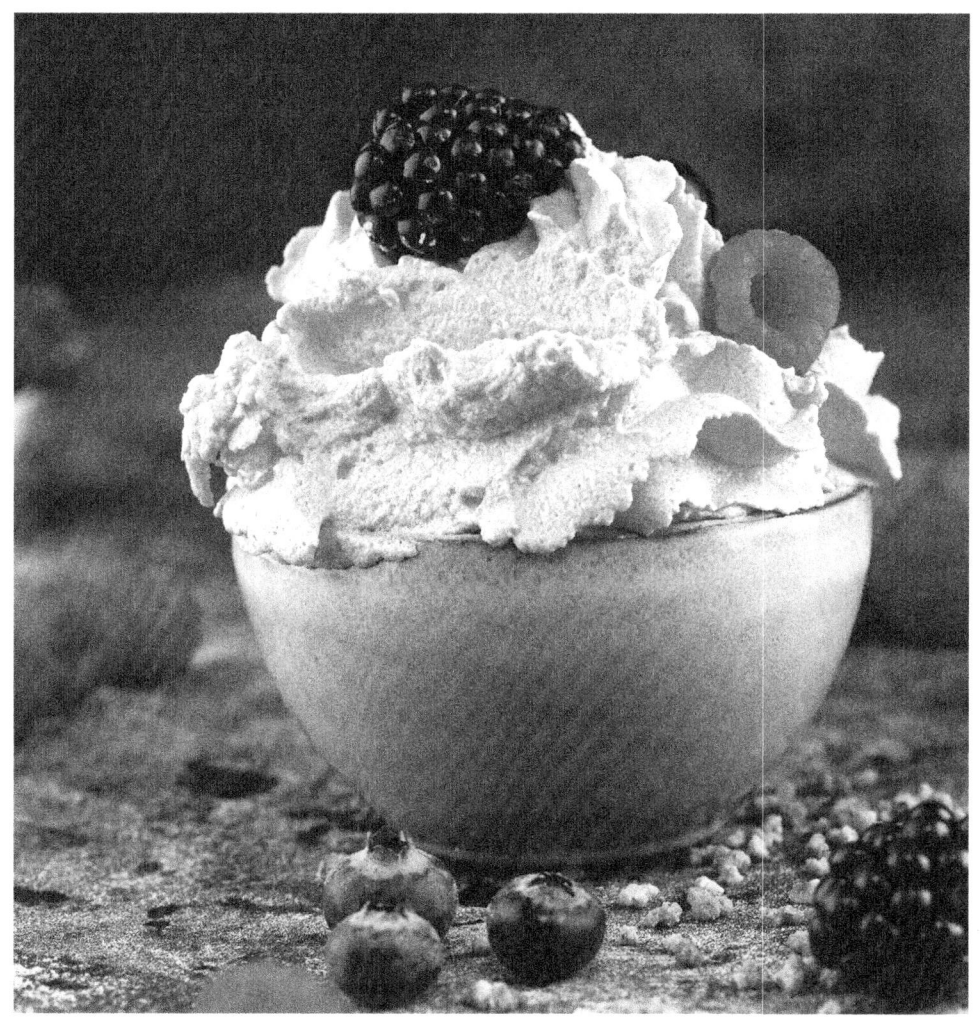

Preparing for Your First Soft-Serve

When you prep for your first soft-serve you will need at least two frozen bananas without the peel. Plus the ingredients listed in one of the 101 luscious recipes you decide to whip up. You'll need to clean the machine before you start, too. So how do you properly clean your frozen treat maker? Read on...

How to Clean Your Frozen Treat Maker

Remove the Full Chute Assembly from the base of your frozen treat maker. Take the full chute assembly apart. Place all of the individual parts in hot, mild soapy water. Clean only the full chute assembly; do not submerge the base of the machine in water. Wash the assembly parts by hand with a soft cloth or sponge. Rinse with cool water. The manufacturer usually recommends that you "not use any abrasive cleaning products"—especially those not fit for human consumption. Wipe the parts down with a clean towel, or dry them overnight on a drying rack.

How to Make Your First Soft-Serve

Gather the ingredients for your first recipe. If you just want to try bananas, break the bananas into pieces so they will fit into the machine. Put a bowl under the front of your frozen treat maker. Turn the machine on. Push the banana through the machine using the plunger. In seconds you will have delicious soft-serve "ice cream."

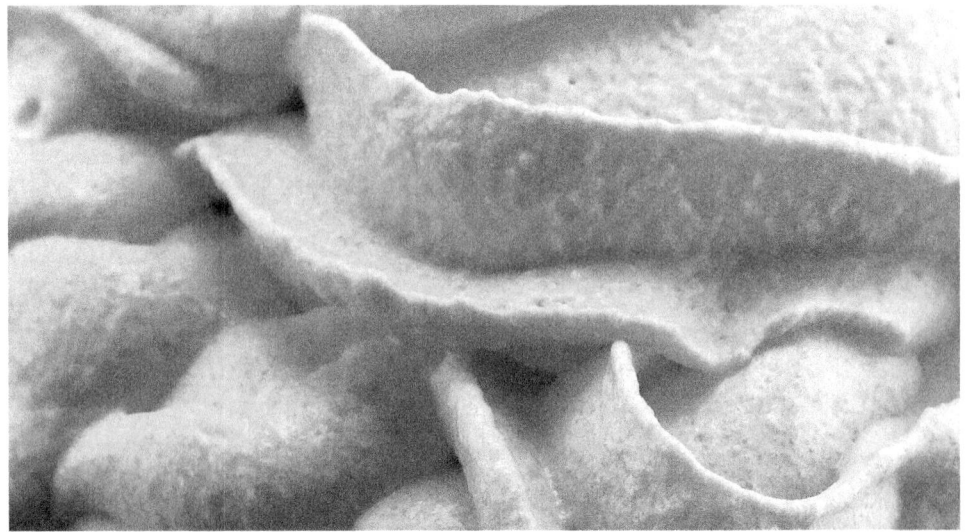

How to Maintain Your Frozen Treat Maker

Clean your frozen treat maker after every use. Only use your frozen treat maker for its intended use as described in the manual. While your frozen treat maker is kid friendly, it's not a toy; be sure to supervise children whenever they are using the machine.

How to Store Your Frozen Treat Maker

Be sure the entire machine is completely dry, including all of the full chute assembly parts. Be careful about any moisture in or around said parts as it can grow mold, so wipe it down well. Put the appliance back together. Place the appliance back in its box and store at room temperature, frost-free, dry place, out of reach of kids.

CHAPTER 5
Pro Tips to Make Perfect Soft-Serve Dessert

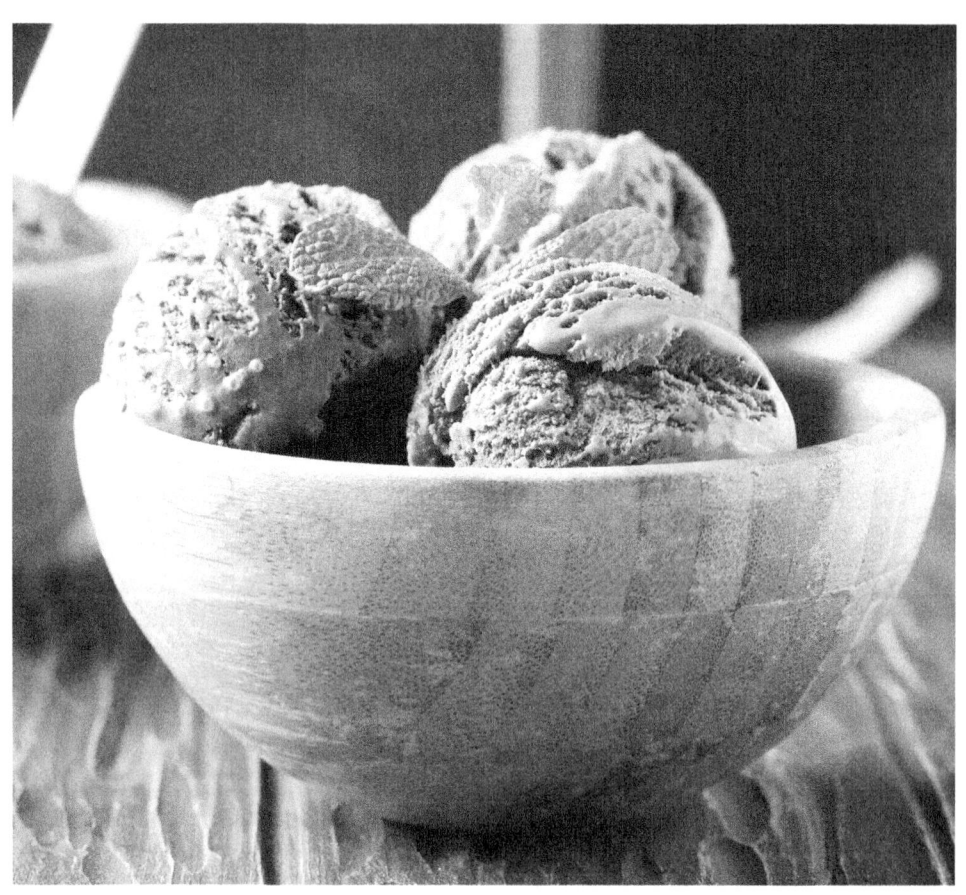

The Best Fruit to Use

The best bananas to use in your frozen treat maker are overripe, brown-spotted bananas. Especially if you are whipping up one of the delicious 101 recipes. An overripe banana is sweeter and takes on the other flavors for a tastier experience! To freeze, peel the bananas and discard the peel. Place the bananas in an air-tight container. Freeze for 24 hours and up three months. After three months your bananas may still keep but can begin to get freezer burn. Once they crystallize, or a layer of ice forms, it will cause your soft-serve to taste stale. Time to freeze some fresh, ripe bananas.

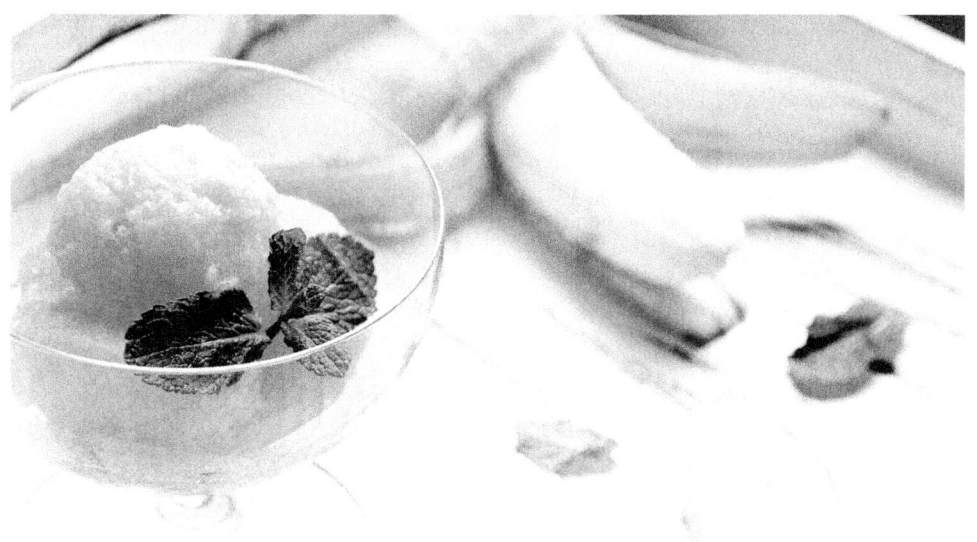

How to Prep Fresh Fruit & Freeze

To prep all other fruit that has a peel, like Kiwi, follow the instructions above. Some fruit, like oranges, may need to be deseeded before freezing. Be conscious of the fruit you are using. For instance, strawberries will require the tops to be removed. Unlike juicing you want to use the meat of the fruit but not stems or leaves. All other fruit should be rinsed thoroughly and lightly dried on a paper towel before freezing to eliminate excess water that can cause freezer burn.

Best Time to Freeze Fruit

The best time to freeze fruit for use in your frozen treat maker is at optimum ripeness. For instance bananas should be over-ripe and spotted, but not black. Strawberries should be dark red, but not moldy. Cantaloupe should be dark orange but not mushy, and so on.

Tips for Adding Fruit

Let your fruit defrost outside of the freezer for 10 minutes before you start using your frozen treat maker. This will yield the best tasting ice cream and you will get more of the fruit into the bowl. You will also be less likely lose your first banana.

What to Do if You Lose Your First Banana?

Sometimes when you make fruit based frozen soft-serve the first banana will almost completely disappear and not reappear as ice cream in your bowl. If this happens, simply remove the full chute assembly from the front of your frozen treat maker. Next, twist the black, circular base piece off of the chute. Remove the white cone inside the base of the chute. Voila! There is your first banana. Simply spoon it into your bowl along with the additional soft-serve. This is likely due to the fruit not being defrosted long enough. Simply wait another five to ten minutes when defrosting your fruits before you make your ice cream for a total of 15 minutes defrost time.

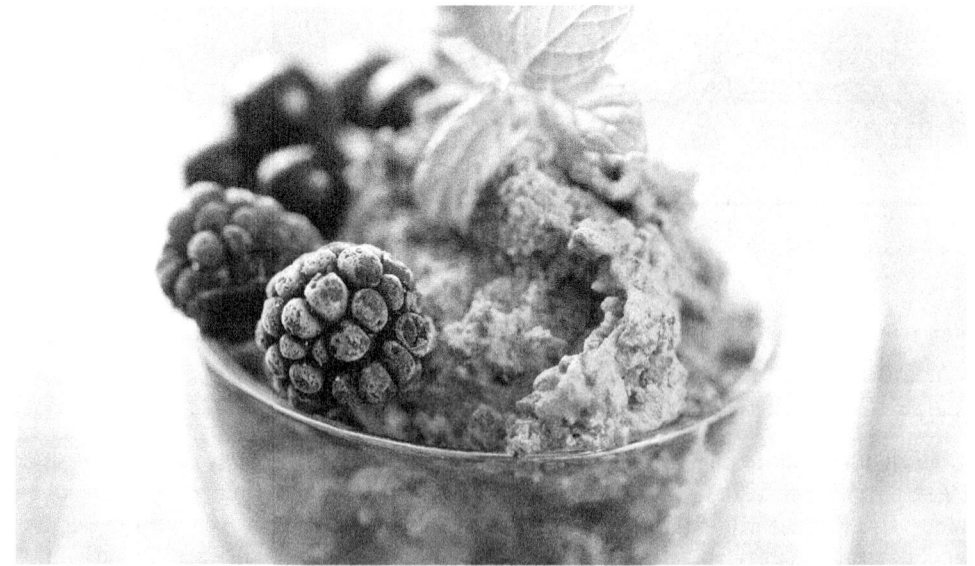

The Best Dish to Use to Catch Fruit Based Soft-Serve

When catching your fruit based soft-serve, a bowl twice the size of your intended serving is optimal—especially for mixing up recipes. If making more than one serving, a metal mixing bowl is the best option because it will keep the soft-serve super cool until you are ready to divvy the decadent treat up into individual servings.

CHAPTER 6
How to Store Your Soft-Serve Desserts

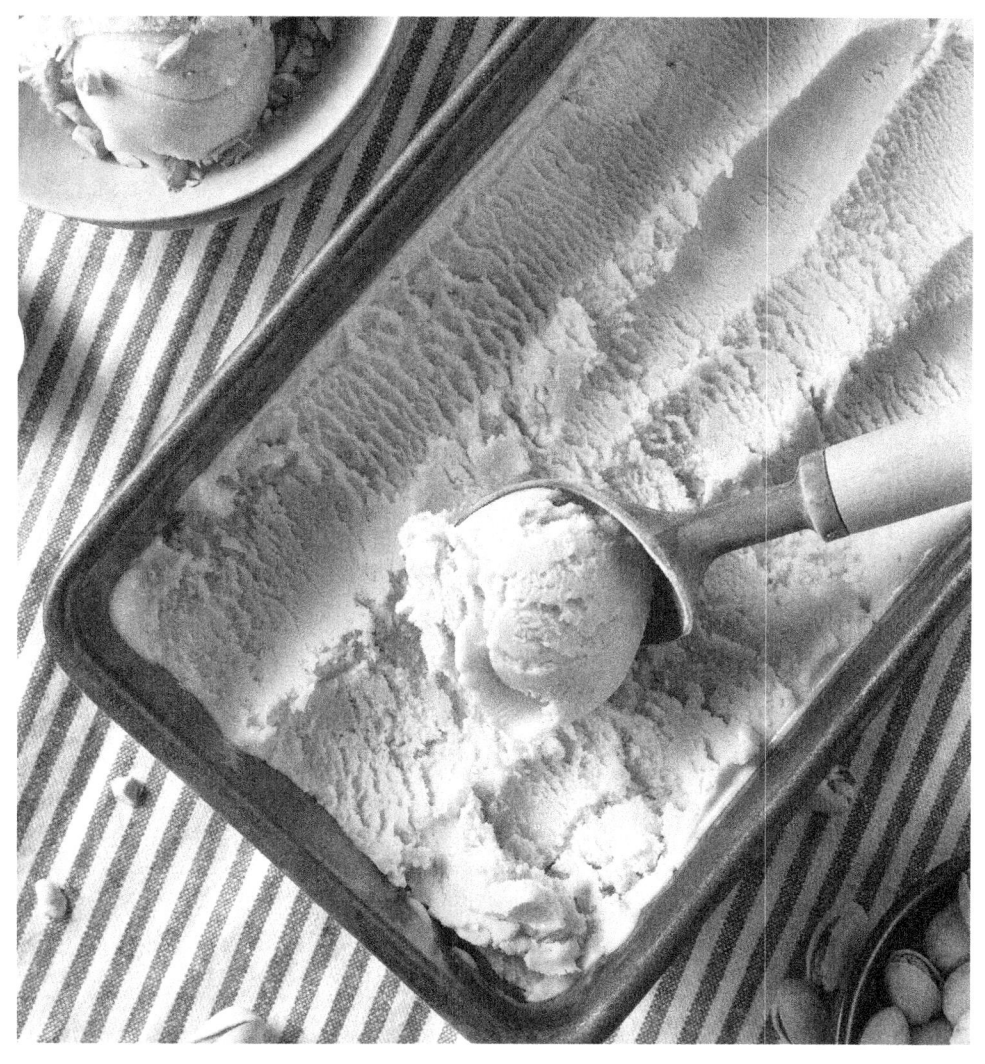

The Best Container to Use for Storage

The best container to use for storing all of your delicious fruit based frozen treats is a freezer-safe, shallow, airtight container. Reusable, rectangular plastic containers are great, as well as stackable, to keep your freezer organized. Simply clean and rinse your container. Dry very well, as excess water can cause freezer burn. Place your soft-serve in the container and freeze. For individual servings, store in styrofoam cups with a plastic lid. You can even make fruit based pops for the whole family using a popsicle mold.

How Long Can I Keep My Frozen Dessert?

You can keep your delicious frozen soft-serve dessert for up to three weeks. If it begins to crystalize and form freezer burn, your ice cream is ready to be thrown out and it's time to whip up a new batch.

How to Store Your Frozen Dessert

Check the temperature of your freezer. Ice cream is best stored at 0 degrees Fahrenheit or below. Simply adjust the temperature of your freezer as needed.

Place your airtight container of delicious soft-serve dessert in the back of your freezer. This keeps it from changing temperature, so it will keep longer. Keeping it in the door or in the front of the freezer exposes your frozen treat to warm elements that can cause freezer burn.

Tips & Tricks to Keep Out Freezer Burn

Start by making sure your container is completely dry. Don't let your soft-serve dessert melt either, freeze it as soon as you make it. Place a layer of cling wrap firmly over the top of your container, then place the lid on tight over the layer of cling film.

CHAPTER 7
Recipes

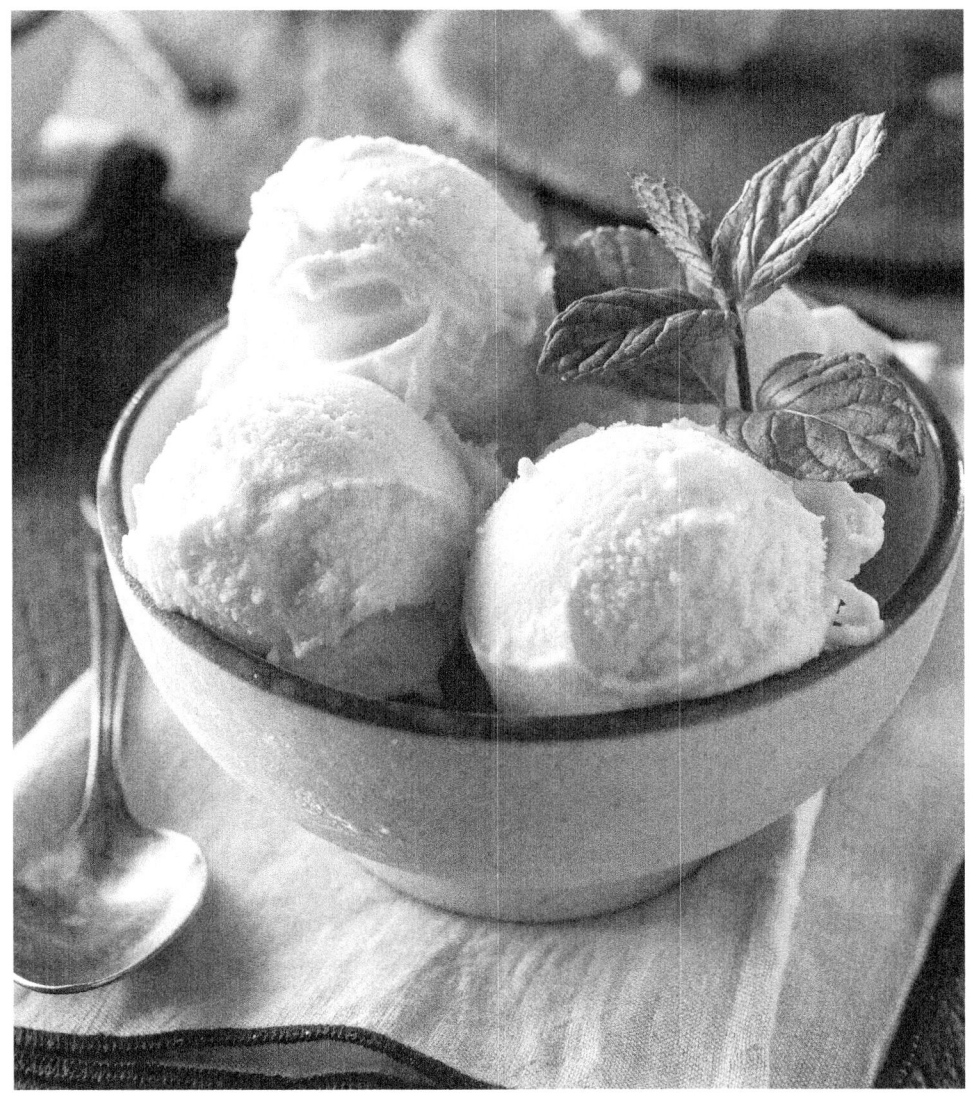

Vanilla Ice Cream

Nothing beats a classic, like creamy vanilla soft-serve when it comes to the perfect dessert. Cool down with a creamy bowl, top it with fresh fruit or your favorite sugar-free sauce like chocolate, caramel, or strawberry for a super-sweet treat.

YIELD: 5 SERVINGS | PREP TIME: 5 MINUTES | COOK TIME: 5 MINUTES

INGREDIENTS:

- 6 frozen bananas, peeled
- 1/4 cup vanilla soy milk
- 1/2 cup soy-based plain yogurt
- 1 tablespoon honey
- 1/4 teaspoon pure vanilla extract
- 1/2 teaspoon pink Himalayan salt, crushed

INSTRUCTIONS:

1. Place a large mixing bowl under the fruit chute.
2. Push frozen bananas through the chute.
3. Add honey, salt, soy milk, frozen yogurt and frozen vanilla extract.
4. Mix until smooth.
5. Spoon into individual bowls.
6. Freeze leftovers in an airtight container.

Nutritional Info: Calories: 163, Sodium: 257mg, Dietary Fiber: 3.7g, Total Fat: 1.0g, Total Carbs: 38.2g, Protein: 3.3g.

Marmalade Ice Cream

Take a step into British summertime with a creamy bowl of bittersweet Marmalade Ice Cream. A scrumptious treat for a fall day, this delicious dessert is one that pairs perfectly with toasted marshmallow or a bottle of craft beer.

YIELD: 6 SERVINGS | PREP TIME: 5 MINUTES | COOK TIME: 3-5 MINUTES

INGREDIENTS:

- 9 frozen bananas, peeled
- 1/4 cup almond milk
- 1/2 cup soy-based yogurt
- 1 tablespoon honey
- 1 tablespoon pure vanilla extract
- 1/2 cup orange marmalade

INSTRUCTIONS:

1. Place a large mixing bowl under the fruit chute.
2. Push frozen bananas through the chute using the plunger.
3. Add almond milk, yogurt, honey, and vanilla extract to the mixing bowl.
4. Mix together until smooth.
5. Place a one-inch layer of the soft-serve into a rectangular airtight container or cake tin.
6. Spoon teaspoons of orange marmalade sporadically onto the smoothed over soft-serve. **This will give your ice cream a marbled effect.
7. Add another one-inch layer of soft-serve and repeat spooning marmalade.
8. Add a final layer of ice cream.
9. Spoon into individual bowls.
10. Freeze leftovers in an airtight container.

Nutritional Info: Calories: 260, Sodium: 36mg, Dietary Fiber: 4.8g, Total Fat: 1.0g, Total Carbs: 63.2g, Protein: 3.5g.

Bourbon Ice Cream

Whip up a yummy southern-style treat with this delicious recipe that combines the velvet of bourbon with creamy vanilla. While this might not be the first thing when you think of healthy desserts, this sweet treat will blow your foodie mind.

YIELD: 5 SERVINGS | PREP TIME: 10 MINUTES | COOK TIME: 5 MINUTES

INGREDIENTS:

- 6 frozen bananas, peeled
- 1 cup soy-based yogurt
- 1 teaspoon pure vanilla extract
- 1/4 cup brown sugar substitute
- 3 tablespoons bourbon

INSTRUCTIONS:

1. Place a large mixing bowl under the fruit chute.
2. Push frozen bananas through the chute.
3. Add yogurt, vanilla extract, brown sugar, and bourbon to the mixing bowl.
4. Mix together until smooth.
5. Spoon into individual bowls.
6. Freeze leftovers in an airtight container.

Nutritional Info: Calories: 231, Sodium: 36mg, Dietary Fiber: 3.7g, Total Fat: 1.1g, Total Carbs: 45.5g, Protein: 4.3g.

Mojito Sorbet

One crisp, refreshing dessert Mojito Sorbet will make your taste buds pop with the taste of sweet lime and fresh mint. Imagine setting sail on the high seas after every bite of this absolutely lush soft-serve that packs a rum punch.

YIELD: 4 SERVINGS | PREP TIME: 5 MINUTES | COOK TIME: 5 MINUTES

INGREDIENTS:

- 6 frozen bananas, peeled
- 5 sprigs of mint, chopped
- 3 tablespoons freshly-squeezed lime juice
- 3 tablespoons dark rum
- 1 teaspoon lime zest

INSTRUCTIONS:

1. Place a large mixing bowl under the fruit chute.
2. Push frozen bananas through the chute.
3. Add mint, frozen lime juice, frozen rum and zest to the mixing bowl.
4. Mix until smooth.
5. Spoon into individual bowls.
6. Freeze leftovers in an airtight container.

Nutritional Info: Calories: 193, Sodium: 7mg, Dietary Fiber: 5.7g, Total Fat: 0.7g, Total Carbs: 43.5g, Protein: 2.5g.

Lime-Basil Sorbet

A delicious Italian-inspired sorbet, this fresh little treat boasts of tart with a spicy kick. Enjoy this tantalizing treat on the hottest of days, or to cleanse your palate on a family-style night of wine tasting and tapas with friends.

YIELD: 4 SERVINGS | PREP TIME: 5 MINUTES | COOK TIME: 5 MINUTES

INGREDIENTS:

- 6 frozen bananas, peeled
- 1/2 cup freshly-squeezed lime juice
- 2 tablespoons lime zest
- 3 tablespoons fresh basil, chopped
- Sprig of fresh basil to garnish for parties

INSTRUCTIONS:

1. Place a large mixing bowl under the fruit chute.
2. Push the frozen bananas through the chute.
3. Add lime juice, zest and basil to the mixing bowl.
4. Mix until well-blended.
5. Spoon into individual bowls.
6. Freeze leftovers in an airtight container.

Nutritional Info: Calories: 161, Sodium: 2mg, Dietary Fiber: 5.0g, Total Fat: 0.6g, Total Carbs: 41.4g, Protein: 2.1g.

Zucchini-Lemon Sorbet

When it comes to finding ways to sneak a serving of vegetables into your favorite treat, this is the way to go! Packed with protein, vitamin A, K and B6—this is seriously one healthy, yet "Oh! So very delicious" treat.

YIELD: 4 SERVINGS | PREP TIME: 5 MINUTES | COOK TIME: 5 MINUTES

INGREDIENTS:

- 3 frozen bananas, peeled
- 2 frozen zucchinis, peeled
- 1/4 cup lemon juice
- 1 tablespoon lemon zest

INSTRUCTIONS:

1. Place a large mixing bowl under the fruit chute.
2. Push the frozen bananas through the chute.
3. Push the zucchini through the chute.
4. Add the lemon juice and zest to the mixing bowl.
5. Mix until well-blended.
6. Spoon into individual bowls, and freeze leftovers in an airtight container.

Nutritional Info: Calories: 99, Sodium: 14mg, Dietary Fiber: 3.5g, Total Fat: 0.6g, Total Carbs: 24.1g, Protein: 2.3g.

Raspberry-Campari Sorbet

Mix up a taste of Italian summertime with this after-dinner drink inspired sorbet. A delicious palate cleanser this treat is perfect for wine tastings, warm evenings when the sun goes down, and for a healthy treat with an Italian kick.

YIELD: 2-4 SERVINGS | PREP TIME: 5 MINUTES | COOK TIME: 5 MINUTES

INGREDIENTS:

- 5 cups frozen raspberries
- 2 tablespoons honey
- 3 tablespoons Campari
- 1 teaspoon fresh-squeezed orange juice
- 1/2 teaspoon fresh orange zest
- 1/4 teaspoon kosher salt
- 1/2 teaspoon fresh lemon juice

INSTRUCTIONS:

1. Place a large mixing bowl under the fruit chute.
2. Push the frozen raspberries through the chute.
3. Add honey, Campari, orange juice & zest, lemon juice, and salt to the mixing bowl.
4. Mix until well-blended.
5. Spoon into individual bowls.
6. Freeze leftovers in an airtight container.

Nutritional Info: Calories: 192.3, Sodium: 197mg, Dietary Fiber: 13.4g, Total Fat: 1.3g, Total Carbs: 40.5g, Protein: 2.5g.

Pink Grapefruit Sorbet

Want a guilt-free decadent way to eat grapefruit for breakfast? Whip up some super-smooth grapefruit sorbet. Top it with milled flaxseed, almonds, and granola for the perfect energetic morning treat.

YIELD: 2 SERVINGS | PREP TIME: 15 MINUTES | 24 HOURS FOR FREEZING | COOK TIME: 3 MINUTES

INGREDIENTS:

6 frozen grapefruits, peeled

INSTRUCTIONS:

1. Prep the grapefruit by cutting each in half; peel and deseed. Make sure all of the rind (hard skin) is separated from the fruit.
2. Freeze all of the fruit in an airtight container overnight.
3. When you're ready to make the soft-serve, place a large mixing bowl under the fruit chute.
4. Push the frozen grapefruit spears through the chute using the plunger.
5. Mix the soft-serve together until smooth.
6. Spoon into individual bowls, and freeze leftovers in an airtight container.

Nutritional Info: Calories: 123, Sodium: 0mg, Dietary Fiber: 4.2g, Total Fat: 0.4g, Total Carbs: 31.0g, Protein: 2.4g.

Blueberry Cheesecake Ice Cream

When it comes to healthy eating you might crave all those decadent desserts you enjoyed before but can't bring yourself to cheat on your newfound lifestyle. Have no fear. This amazingly creamy soft-serve will really hit the sweet spot!

YIELD: 4-5 SERVINGS | PREP TIME: 5 MINUTES | COOK TIME: 15 MINUTES

INGREDIENTS:

- 6 cups frozen blueberries
- 1 cup vanilla soy-based yogurt
- 1 tablespoon honey
- 1 teaspoon pure vanilla extract
- 8 ounces vegan cream cheese

INSTRUCTIONS:

1. Set the vegan cream cheese out on the counter to come to room temperature for at least 8 hours.
2. Whip the cheese, using an electric mixer, in a large mixing bowl until it is a smooth, creamy texture.
3. Place the mixing bowl with whipped cheese under the fruit chute.
4. Push frozen blueberries through the fruit chute.
5. Add yogurt, vanilla extract, and honey to the mixing bowl.
6. Mix together until smooth.
7. Spoon into individual bowls.
8. Freeze leftovers in an airtight container.

Nutritional Info: Calories: 182, Sodium: 68mg, Dietary Fiber: 4.2g, Total Fat: 1.8g, Total Carbs: 35.4g, Protein: 6.7g.

Almond Nougat Mousse Ice Cream

Nothing beats creamy vanilla mousse laced with decadent nougat made from almonds and as a healthy treat - you'll want to keep a gallon of this in the refrigerator for those days you really want to quench your sweet tooth.

YIELD: 8 SERVINGS | PREP TIME: 2 HOURS 20 MINUTES | COOK TIME: 15 MINUTES

INGREDIENTS:

- 9 frozen bananas, peeled
- 1/3 cup raw almonds, roughly chopped
- 1 cup vanilla flavored soy-based yogurt
- 1 teaspoon vanilla extract
- 1/2 teaspoon almond extract
- Pinch of pink Himalayan salt

Nougat Ingredients:
- 2 large egg whites
- 1/3 cup honey
- 1/2 cup brown sugar substitute

INSTRUCTIONS:

Nougat:

1. Pour soy-based yogurt, vanilla extract and almond extract into a large mixing bowl. Whisk until it forms soft peaks. Place in the refrigerator to chill for 2 hours.
2. Heat a medium saucepan on medium to medium-high heat.
3. Pour in 1/4 cup of the brown sugar and melt before adding the next 1/4 cup of brown sugar. Do not stir; swirl the pan to prevent burning whilst melting the sugar.
4. Once melted, stir in the chopped almonds and pour on the parchment paper lined cookie sheet to cool.
5. Whip the egg whites in a second mixing bowl until soft peaks form.

6. Heat the 1/4 cup of honey in a small saucepan over medium heat until it thins. Slowly add the honey to the whites. Whip with an electric mixer on low.
7. Once all the honey is incorporated, increase the mixer speed to high; when the bowl is no longer warm and stiff peaks have formed your meringue is ready.
8. Chop up the almond pieces on the cookie sheet.

Soft-Serve:

1. Remove the mixing bowl of yogurt from the refrigerator and place under the fruit chute.
2. Push the bananas through the chute.
3. Fold the meringue and nut pieces into the mix and stir until smooth.
4. Spoon into individual bowls.

Nutritional Info: Calories: 272, Sodium: 39mg, Dietary Fiber: 4.0g, Total Fat: 3.0g, Total Carbs: 56.1g, Protein: 6.1g.

Apple Sorbet

If you love apples, this refreshing dessert is just what the doctor ordered! Packed with deliciously sweet apples and a hint of tangy lemon, apple sorbet the perfect healthy snack for the apple lover at heart.

YIELD: 3-5 SERVINGS | PREP TIME: 5 MINUTES | COOK TIME: 5 MINUTES

INGREDIENTS:

- 5 frozen apples, peeled, cored and deseeded
- 3 tablespoons fresh pressed apple juice
- 1/2 teaspoon lemon juice

INSTRUCTIONS:

1. Place a large mixing bowl under the fruit chute and push the apples through.
2. Add apple and lemon juice.
3. Stir until smooth.
4. Spoon into individual bowls and freeze leftovers in an airtight container.

Nutritional Info: Calories: 165, Sodium: 3mg, Dietary Fiber: 7.4g, Total Fat: 0.6g, Total Carbs: 43.7g, Protein: 0.8g.

Mango Tango

A tangy tart treat packed with vitamin C might be just what the doctor ordered for a tantalizing dessert on a warm day. Mango Tango sorbet is loaded with tangy taste for one delicious way to enjoy a bowl full of healthy essential vitamins.

YIELD: 4 SERVINGS | PREP TIME: 5 MINUTES | COOK TIME: 5 MINUTES

INGREDIENTS:

1 bag frozen mango
1 frozen orange, peeled and seeded
5 frozen tangerines, peeled and seeded
3 tablespoons lime juice
1 tablespoon lime zest

INSTRUCTIONS:

1. Place a large mixing bowl under the fruit chute.
2. Push the frozen mango, orange and tangerines through the fruit chute.
3. Add the lime juice and zest to the mixing bowl.
4. Mix until well-blended.
5. Spoon into individual bowls, and freeze leftovers in an airtight container.

Nutritional Info: Calories: 121, Sodium: 8mg, Dietary Fiber: 3.4g, Total Fat: 0.3g, Total Carbs: 31.0g, Protein: 1.7g.

Pumpkin Pie Ice Cream

Kick things up a notch for the holidays with this delicious pumpkin pie ice cream that is literally "out of this world". While this ice cream is great when you first whip it up, it's even more delicious once the flavors set in overnight. Enjoy it on a cool fall evening with a latte or with family and friends for an after dinner dessert.

YIELD: 4-6 SERVINGS | PREP TIME: 7 MINUTES | COOK TIME: 24 HOURS

INGREDIENTS:

- 12 frozen bananas, peeled
- 1 cup vanilla soy-based yogurt
- 1 teaspoon ground cinnamon
- 1 teaspoon allspice
- 1 can pumpkin puree
- 2 graham crackers per bowl, crushed (optional topping)

INSTRUCTIONS:

1. Place a large mixing bowl under the fruit chute and push the bananas through.
2. Add soy-based yogurt, cinnamon, allspice and pumpkin puree to the bowl.
3. Stir until smooth.
4. Place soft-serve in an airtight container and freeze for 24 hours.
5. Top with crushed graham crackers for the ultimate pumpkin pie taste!

Nutritional Info: Calories: 274, Sodium: 45mg, Dietary Fiber: 7.7g, Total Fat: 2.2g, Total Carbs: 62.9g, Protein: 7.2g.

Pineapple Sorbet

For the pineapple lover at heart, this creamy, decadent dessert is just the thing to quench your thirst. Cool down with a bowl of this super-easy recipe and freeze some extra for those day when you just need a frozen pineapple treat.

YIELD: 2 SERVINGS | PREP TIME: 5 MINUTES | COOK TIME: 3-5 MINUTES

INGREDIENTS:

1 small bag of frozen pineapple chunks or 1 small pineapple, peeled, cored and frozen

INSTRUCTIONS:

1. Put frozen bananas through the chute. Using the plunger, push the pineapple down the chute.
2. Push frozen pineapple through the chute.
3. Mix the soft-serve together until smooth.
4. Spoon into individual bowls.

Nutritional Info: Calories: 41, Sodium: 1mg, Dietary Fiber: 1.1g, Total Fat: 0.1g, Total Carbs: 10.8g, Protein: 0.4g.

Raspberry and Redcurrant Sorbet

For a fruity treat that is so very simple to make, look no further than a combination of raspberries and redcurrant. This palate cleansing sorbet is perfect for dinner parties or served with vanilla rolled wafers.

YIELD: 2-4 SERVINGS | PREP TIME: 5 MINUTES | COOK TIME: 5 MINUTES

INGREDIENTS:

- 5 cups frozen raspberries
- 2 cups frozen redcurrants, destemmed

INSTRUCTIONS:

1. Place a large mixing bowl under the fruit chute and push the raspberries and redcurrants through.
2. Stir until smooth to blend the flavors.
3. Spoon into individual bowls and freeze leftovers in an airtight container.

Nutritional Info: Calories: 160, Sodium: 3mg, Dietary Fiber: 20.0g, Total Fat: 2.0g, Total Carbs: 36.7g, Protein: 3.7g.

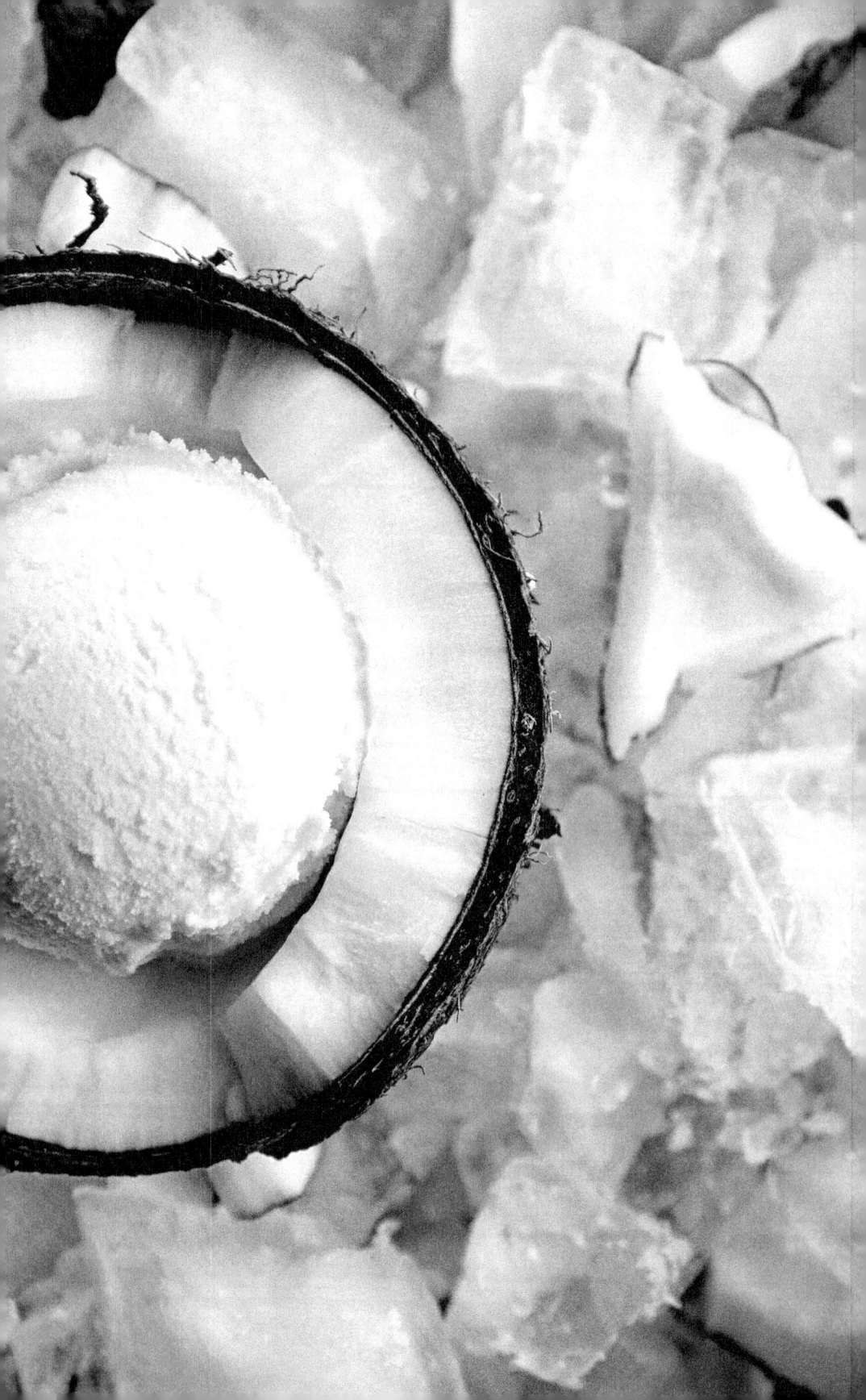

Coconut Caramel Ice Cream

Nothing quite beats a sweet bowl of creamy coconut soft-serve laced with rich caramel when it comes to one lush dessert combination. This dessert is so simple, you might just make a whole gallon to enjoy as an after-dinner dessert all week long.

YIELD: 2-4 SERVINGS | PREP TIME: 5 MINUTES | COOK TIME: 5 MINUTES

INGREDIENTS:

- 6 frozen bananas, peeled
- 1 bag fresh frozen coconut
- 1 teaspoon pure coconut extract
- 1 teaspoon brown sugar substitute
- 2 teaspoons pure vanilla extract
- 1/4 cup calorie free caramel sauce

INSTRUCTIONS:

1. Place a large mixing bowl under the fruit chute and push the bananas and coconut through.
2. Add coconut extract, vanilla extract and brown sugar substitute to the mixing bowl.
3. Mix until smooth.
4. Spoon into individual bowls.
5. Top with caramel sauce.
6. Freeze leftovers in an airtight container.

Nutritional Info: Calories: 294, Sodium: 78mg, Dietary Fiber: 6.6g, Total Fat: 7.3g, Total Carbs: 58.4g, Protein: 2.9g.

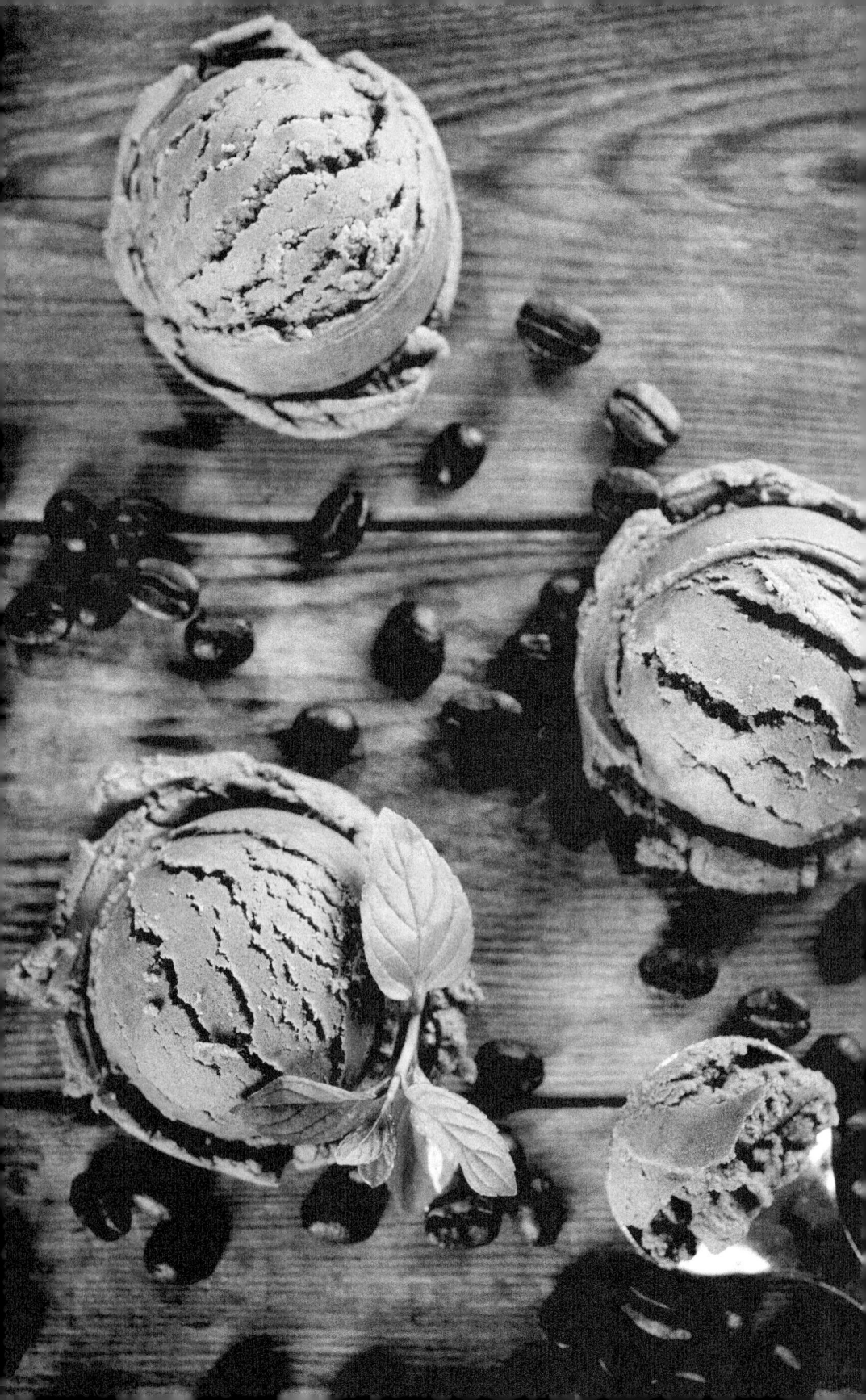

Chocolate-Coffee Ice Cream

Taste the subtle flavor of coffee in your smooth frozen fruit treat. This dessert, having caffeine, might not be everyone's favorite but the rich chocolate taste will surely entice your appetite.

YIELD: 2-4 SERVINGS | PREP TIME: 2 HOURS 5 MINUTES | COOK TIME: 5 MINUTES

INGREDIENTS:

- 9 frozen bananas, peeled
- 1 cup plain soy-based yogurt
- 2 tablespoons coffee
- 1 tablespoon brown sugar substitute
- 1/4 cup chocolate covered espresso beans, chopped

INSTRUCTIONS:

1. Whip the soy-based yogurt with coffee and brown sugar substitute.
2. Place in the refrigerator for 2 hours to set.
3. Place a large mixing bowl under the fruit chute and push the bananas through.
4. Fold the coffee yogurt into the mixing bowl.
5. Mix until smooth.
6. Spoon into individual bowls and top with chocolate covered espresso beans.
7. Freeze leftovers in an airtight container.

Nutritional Info: Calories: 297, Sodium: 22mg, Dietary Fiber: 7.1g, Total Fat: 2.0g, Total Carbs: 66.5g, Protein: 8.8g.

Brownie Batter No-Churn Ice Cream

Brownie lovers will absolutely go ape for this confectionary filled ice cream that tastes a little like heaven. With brownies folded right into your scrumptious soft-serve this treat is "Oh, so sweet!"

YIELD: 2-4 SERVINGS | PREP TIME: 2 HOURS 5 MINUTES | COOK TIME: 5 MINUTES

INGREDIENTS:

- 9 frozen bananas, peeled
- 1/2 cup vanilla soy-based yogurt
- 1 teaspoon cocoa powder
- 2 gluten free brownies, chopped

INSTRUCTIONS:

1. Whip the soy-based yogurt with cocoa powder
2. Place in the refrigerator for 2 hours to set.
3. Place a large mixing bowl under the fruit chute and push the bananas through.
4. Fold the chocolate yogurt into the soft-serve.
5. Mix until smooth.
6. Add brownie bites and mix delicately.
7. Spoon into individual bowls and freeze leftovers in an airtight container.

Nutritional Info: Calories: 337, Sodium: 63mg, Dietary Fiber: 7.0g, Total Fat: 5.6g, Total Carbs: 69.2g, Protein: 9.5g.

Bananas with Toasted Coconut, Almonds, & Dark Chocolate

For one rich banana filled treat look no further than this super-lush recipe! Simple and decadent, this dessert is great for those days you just want to be bad, but still keep your diet super-food healthy.

YIELD: 3 SERVINGS | PREP TIME: 5 MINUTES | COOK TIME: 5 MINUTES

INGREDIENTS:

- 9 frozen bananas, peeled
- 5 tablespoons coconut, toasted
- 3 tablespoons 70-85% dark cacao bar, chopped
- 3 tablespoons almonds, chopped

INSTRUCTIONS:

1. Place a large mixing bowl under the fruit chute and push the bananas through.
2. Spoon into individual bowls.
3. Top each serving with toasted coconut, chocolate chunks and almonds.
4. Freeze leftovers in an airtight container.

Nutritional Info: Calories: 391, Sodium: 6mg, Dietary Fiber: 12.3g, Total Fat: 7.6g, Total Carbs: 86.3g, Protein: 6.4g.

Red Plum Sorbet

A healthy way to detox, this tart-filled sorbet can be made even more decadent when topped with creamy whipped topping. You'll be sure to savor this one, one delicious healthy bite at a time. Try out this delicious recipe for days you just feel like detoxing.

YIELD: 2-4 SERVINGS | PREP TIME: 5 MINUTES | COOK TIME: 5 MINUTES

INGREDIENTS:

- 9 frozen plums, pitted and quartered
- 1/3 teaspoon cardamom powder
- 3 tablespoons of honey
- 1 teaspoon lemon juice

INSTRUCTIONS:

1. Place a large mixing bowl under the fruit chute and push the plums through.
2. Add cardamom powder, honey and lemon juice to the mixing bowl.
3. Mix until smooth to blend the flavors.
4. Spoon into individual bowls.
5. Freeze leftovers in an airtight container.

Nutritional Info: Calories: 93, Sodium: 1mg, Dietary Fiber: 1.4g, Total Fat: 0.3g, Total Carbs: 24.3g, Protein: 0.8g.

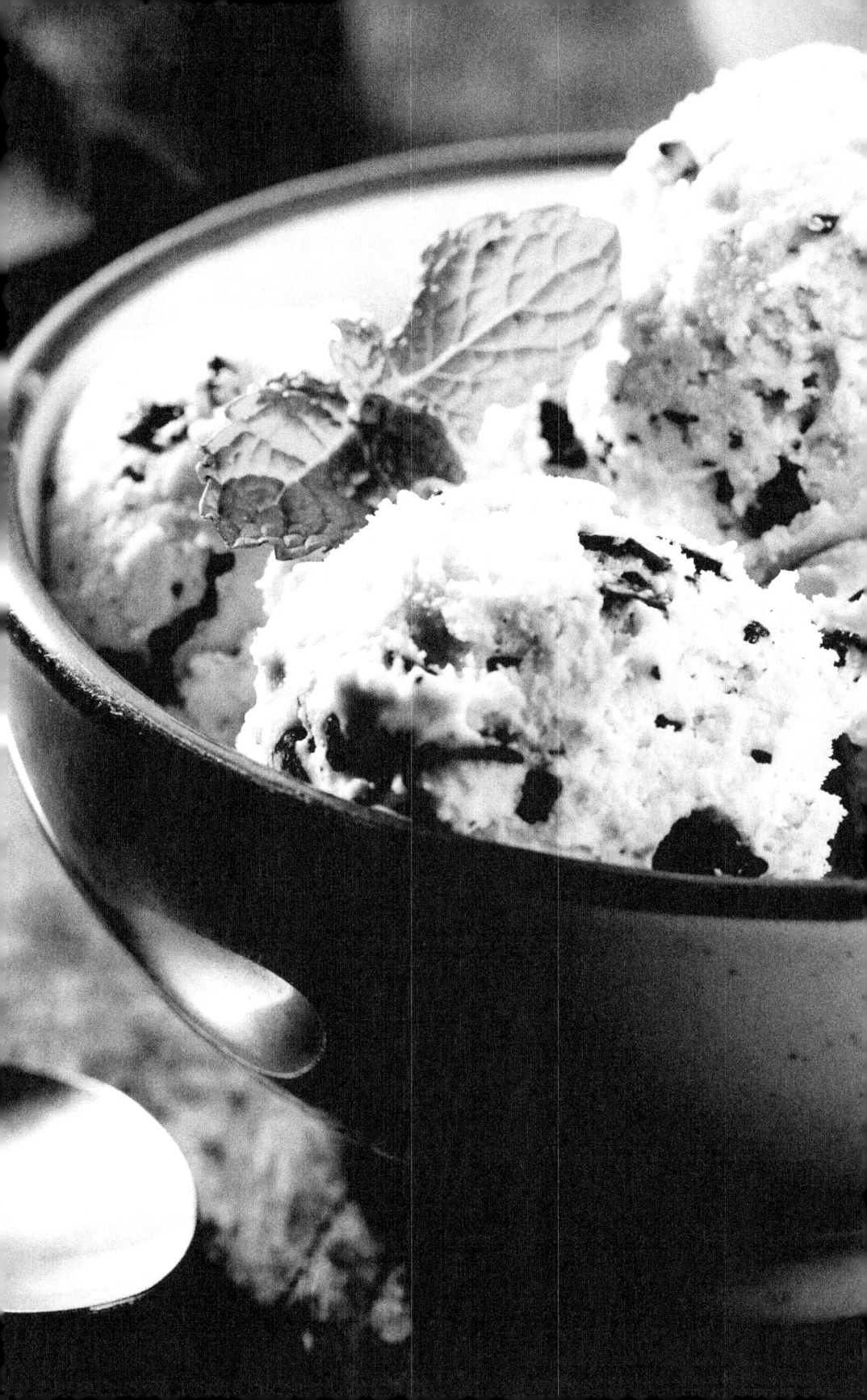

Mint Chocolate Chip Ice Cream

Mint chocolate chip lovers unite! As if we'd leave this creamy, velvet classic out. When it comes to soft-serve, this minty treat is more than a classic dessert—it's packed with antioxidants and serves as a great palate cleanser too!

YIELD: 3 SERVINGS | PREP TIME: 5 MINUTES | COOK TIME: 5 MINUTES

INGREDIENTS:

- 9 frozen bananas, peeled
- 1/2 frozen avocado, peeled and pitted
- 1 tablespoon honey
- 5 mint leaves, chopped
- 1/2 teaspoon mint extract
- 1/3 cup 85% dark cacao bar, chopped

INSTRUCTIONS:

1. Place a large mixing bowl under the fruit chute and push the bananas and avocado through.
2. Add honey, mint, mint extract and dark chocolate chunks to the mixing bowl.
3. Mix until well-blended.
4. Spoon into individual bowls and freeze leftovers in an airtight container.

Nutritional Info: Calories: 434, Sodium: 13mg, Dietary Fiber: 15.6g, Total Fat: 9.1g, Total Carbs: 96.3g, Protein: 6.9g.

Caramelized Pecan Banana "Ice Cream" with Chocolate Hazelnut

Creamy ice cream blended with the crunch of caramelized pecans topped with velvety smooth hazelnut is one super-easy dessert to whip up. This dreamy treat will definitely remind you of southern Italy, so don't be afraid to enjoy it with a slice of biscotti or wafer rounds.

YIELD: 3-5 SERVINGS | PREP TIME: 1 HOUR 15 MINUTES | COOK TIME: 5 MINUTES

INGREDIENTS:

1 cup pecan halves
1-1/2 tablespoons brown sugar substitute
1-1/2 teaspoons water
1/8 teaspoon vanilla
1/8 teaspoon Himalayan salt
12 frozen bananas, peeled
2 tablespoons hazelnut spread

INSTRUCTIONS:

1. Combine brown sugar, water, vanilla, and Himalayan salt in a mixing bowl.
2. Stir and set aside.
3. Heat a medium-large saucepan over medium heat and toast pecans for 3 minutes, stirring often to prevent burning.
4. Quickly fold the sugar mixture, set aside, into the pan.
5. Stir well for 10-15 seconds; immediately remove from heat and pour onto a parchment lined baking sheet to cool for 1 hour.
6. Place a large mixing bowl under the fruit chute and push the bananas through.
7. Fold in the caramelized pecans.
8. Spoon into individual bowls and drizzle with hazelnut spread.
9. Freeze leftovers in an airtight container.

Nutritional Info: Calories: 350, Sodium: 61mg, Dietary Fiber: 7.8g, Total Fat: 4.1g, Total Carbs: 78.6g, Protein: 3.7g.

Dark Choco-Peanut Butter Ice Cream

If you love creamy peanut butter surrounded by rich, dark chocolate - this is the soft-serve for you! While the recipe calls for dairy, you can always substitute with your favorite dairy-free versions for a truly decadent vegan style, paleo friendly treat.

YIELD: 3-5 SERVINGS | PREP TIME: 2 HOURS 15 MINUTES | COOK TIME: 5 MINUTES

INGREDIENTS:

- 12 frozen bananas
- 1 cup vanilla soy-based yogurt
- 2 tablespoons cocoa powder
- 1 teaspoon espresso powder
- 1 tablespoon honey
- 2 tablespoons peanut butter, no sugar added
- 3 tablespoons cream cheese, softened to room temperature

INSTRUCTIONS:

1. Whip the soy-based yogurt with cocoa and espresso powder. Place in the refrigerator to set for 2 hours.
2. Mix vegan cream cheese and peanut butter together with an electric mixer until smooth; place in the refrigerator to set with the yogurt.
3. Place a large mixing bowl under the fruit chute and push the bananas through.
4. Fold the chocolate yogurt into the soft-serve and mix until smooth.
5. Add peanut butter cream cheese and mix delicately.
6. Spoon into individual bowls and freeze leftovers in an airtight container.

Nutritional Info: Calories: 363, Sodium: 66mg, Dietary Fiber: 8.4g, Total Fat: 7.5g, Total Carbs: 72.6g, Protein: 10.2g.

Iced Coffee with Banana Ice Cream and Caramel Sauce

Looking for a way to enjoy your coffee and eat it too? Iced coffee with banana ice cream is just the way to indulge. Top it with creamy caramel sauce for the best darn coffee you'll ever have!

YIELD: 1 SERVINGS | PREP TIME: 5 MINUTES | COOK TIME: 3 HOURS 15 MINUTES

INGREDIENTS:

- 3 frozen bananas, peeled
- 1 can full-fat coconut milk
- 1/2 cup fresh brewed coffee
- Water
- Ice

INSTRUCTIONS:

1. Place a kitchen towel in a large saucepan.
2. Add the coconut milk can, unopened, into the pan and cover with water.
3. Bring the water to a boil, cover the pan with a lid, and simmer for three hours; DO NOT let the water boil out. The can will explode if water isn't covering it the entire time it is cooking.
4. Brew fresh coffee and set aside to ice.
5. Remove the can and fold caramel into a large mixing bowl. Whisk in 2 teaspoons of water to make the creamy caramel sauce.
6. Place a second large mixing bowl under the fruit chute and push the bananas through.
7. Add a few cubes of ice to a small rocks style glass and add coffee.
8. Top with banana soft-serve, drizzle with caramel sauce, and enjoy!

Nutritional Info: Calories: 1299, Sodium: 404mg, Dietary Fiber: 9.2g, Total Fat: 27.8g, Total Carbs: 247.3g, Protein: 28.2g.

Berry Ice Cream with Banana Meringue

Swirl in some decadent banana meringue for a cobbler style soft-serve treat without the gluten! Blackberry-blueberry ice cream is packed with the taste of summer that you can enjoy any time of year.

YIELD: 3-5 SERVINGS | PREP TIME: 1 HOUR 5 MINUTES | COOK TIME: 5 MINUTES

INGREDIENTS:

- 2 large egg whites
- 1/3 cup sugar substitute
- 1 teaspoon pure vanilla extract
- 1 very ripe banana, mashed
- 3 cups frozen blackberries
- 2 cups frozen blueberries

INSTRUCTIONS:

1. Whip the egg whites in a mixing bowl until soft peaks form.
2. Add sugar and continue to whip until the mixture starts to thicken.
3. Add mashed banana and vanilla extract; mix well.
4. Place the meringue in the refrigerator to chill for 45 minutes.
5. Place a second mixing bowl under the chute and push the blackberries and blueberries through the chute.
6. Fold the meringue into the soft-serve and swirl with an icing spatula.
7. Spoon into individual bowls.
8. Freeze leftovers in an airtight container.

Nutritional Info: Calories: 151, Sodium: 15mg, Dietary Fiber: 6.6g, Total Fat: 0.7g, Total Carbs: 35.6g, Protein: 3.3g.

Peanut Butter Pretzel Ice Cream

This creamy treat is just the kind of delicious soft-serve that goes great in a waffle cone! Super-easy to whip up in no time, you'll want to make extra to share this super-sweet soft-serve with the ones you love.

YIELD: 4 SERVINGS | PREP TIME: 5 MINUTES | COOK TIME: 5 MINUTES

INGREDIENTS:

- 12 frozen bananas, peeled
- 3 tablespoons all-natural peanut butter, no sugar added
- 1 teaspoon honey
- 1/4 teaspoon pure vanilla extract, frozen
- 1 tablespoon almond milk, frozen
- 1/2 cup gluten-free pretzels, roughly chopped

INSTRUCTIONS:

1. Place a large mixing bowl under the fruit chute and push the bananas through.
2. Add peanut butter, honey, vanilla extract, and almond milk to the mixing bowl.
3. Mix until well-blended.
4. Scoop ice cream into waffle cones and top with pretzel pieces.
5. Freeze leftover soft-serve in an airtight container.

Nutritional Info: Calories: 429, Sodium: 161mg, Dietary Fiber: 10.2g, Total Fat: 8.3g, Total Carbs: 90.8g, Protein: 7.7g.

Spiced Apple Cider Sorbet

If you love drinking warm apple cider by a bonfire or curling up with a warm cup on a holiday night, you will adore this delicious sorbet laced with warm spice and everything nice.

YIELD: 2-4 SERVINGS | PREP TIME: 5 MINUTES | COOK TIME: 5 MINUTES

INGREDIENTS:

- 6 frozen apples, peeled, cored and seeded
- 3 tablespoons fresh pressed apple juice
- 1 teaspoon honey
- 1 teaspoon grated cloves
- 2 teaspoons cinnamon
- 1/2 teaspoon fresh lemon juice
- 2 tablespoons spiced rum

INSTRUCTIONS:

1. Place a large mixing bowl under the fruit chute and push the apples through.
2. Add apple juice, honey, clove, cinnamon, lemon juice and spiced rum to the mixing bowl.
3. Mix until smooth to blend the flavors.
4. Spoon into individual bowls.
5. Freeze leftovers in an airtight container.

Nutritional Info: Calories: 174, Sodium: 4mg, Dietary Fiber: 7.4g, Total Fat: 0.6g, Total Carbs: 41.8g, Protein: 0.8g.

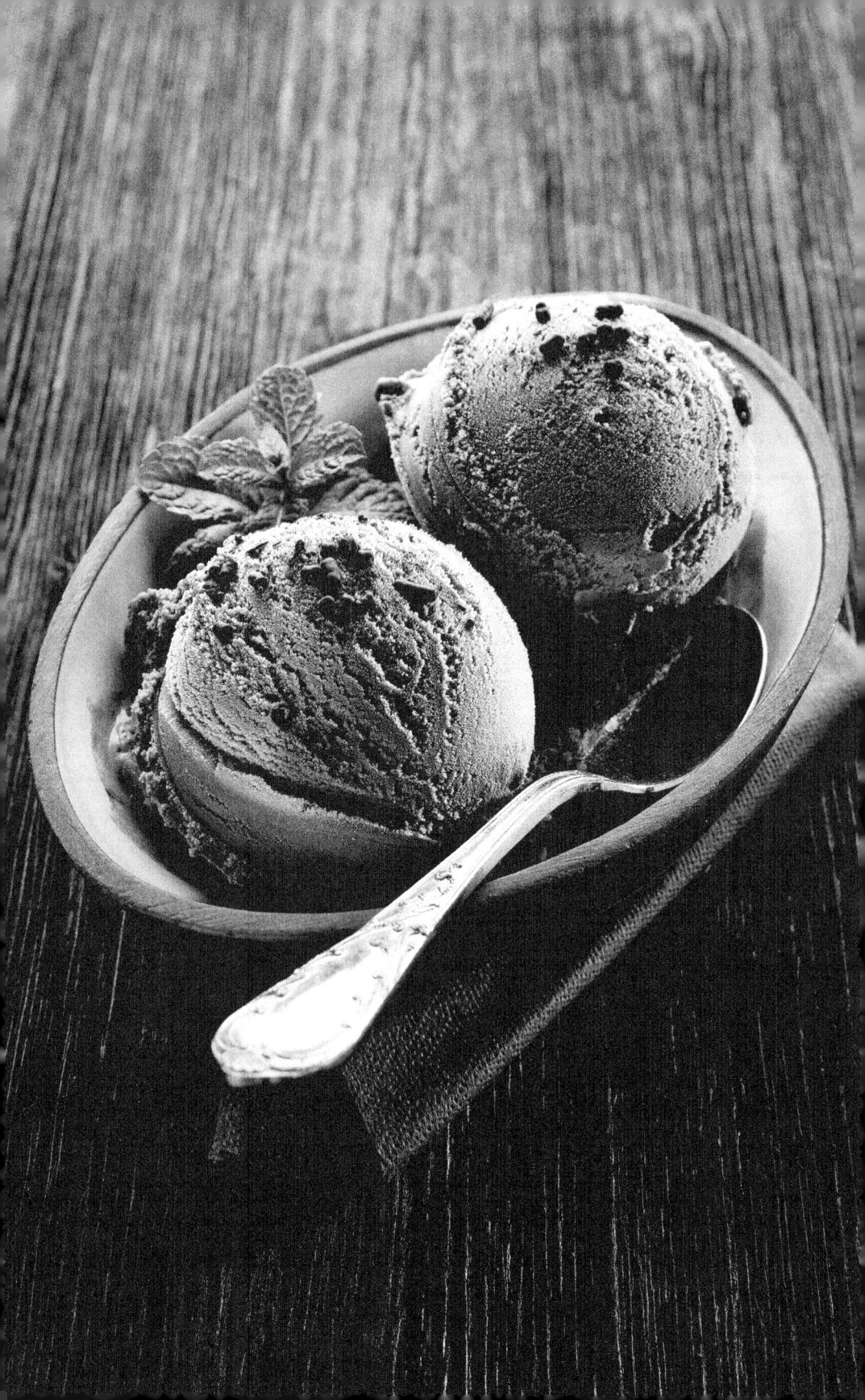

Chocolate Ice Cream

If rich, decadent, creamy chocolate ice cream is your thing—look no further than this delicious recipe. It's packed with everything your chocolate loving heart could desire.

YIELD: 4-6 SERVINGS | PREP TIME: 2 HOURS 5 MINUTES | COOK TIME: 15 MINUTES

INGREDIENTS:

- 12 frozen bananas, peeled
- 2 cups vanilla-soy-based yogurt
- 1/2 cup unsweetened cocoa
- 1/2 cup coffee
- 3 tablespoons vegan cream cheese
- 2 tablespoons honey
- 1/3 cup bittersweet chocolate chips
- 1/3 cup peanut butter chips

INSTRUCTIONS:

1. Pour the soy-based yogurt, unsweetened cocoa and coffee into a large mixing bowl. Whisk until it forms soft peaks. Place in the refrigerator to chill for 2 hours.
2. Place the mixing bowl under the fruit chute and push the bananas through.
3. Add vegan cream cheese, honey, chocolate chips and peanut butter chips to the mix.
4. Stir until smooth. Spoon into single servings and freeze any leftovers.

Nutritional Info: Calories: 435, Sodium: 61mg, Dietary Fiber: 8.8g, Total Fat: 11.4g, Total Carbs: 80.3g, Protein: 12.8g.

Lavender Coconut Ice Cream

De-stress with one cool, scrumptious treat! Soft-serve can help you detox mentally and physically. Lavender is also known for improving blood circulation along with easing pain, so whip up some of this delicious soft-serve to help boost your mood and your energy.

YIELD: 2 SERVINGS | PREP TIME: 5 MINUTES | COOK TIME: 5 MINUTES

INGREDIENTS:

- 6 frozen bananas, peeled
- 1/2 cup coconut flavored soy-based yogurt
- 2 tablespoons lavender flowers, chopped
- 1/2 teaspoon honey

INSTRUCTIONS:

1. Place a large mixing bowl under the fruit chute and push the bananas through.
2. Add yogurt, lavender flowers, and honey to the mixing bowl.
3. Mix until smooth.
4. Scoop ice cream into individual bowls.
5. Freeze leftover soft-serve in an airtight container.

Nutritional Info: Calories: 371.5, Sodium: 46mg, Dietary Fiber: 9.2g, Total Fat: 2.05g, Total Carbs: 88.25g, Protein: 7.5g.

Sugar-free Coconut Vanilla Ice Cream

Keeping it diet friendly when it comes to whipping up sweet treats is so super simple. Especially if you whip up a bowl of sugar-free coconut vanilla ice cream for dessert. This soft-serve is also perfect served with gluten-free animal crackers.

YIELD: 2 SERVINGS | PREP TIME: 5 MINUTES | COOK TIME: 5 MINUTES

INGREDIENTS:

- 6 frozen bananas, peeled
- 3 tablespoons unsweetened coconut milk
- 1 teaspoon pure vanilla extract
- 1/2 teaspoon pure coconut extract
- 1/2 teaspoon sugar substitute (like Stevia)

INSTRUCTIONS:

1. Place a large mixing bowl under the fruit chute and push the bananas through.
2. Add coconut milk, vanilla extract, coconut extract, sugar substitute and mix until smooth.
3. Scoop ice cream into individual bowls.
4. Freeze leftover soft-serve in an airtight container.

Nutritional Info: Calories: 376, Sodium: 7mg, Dietary Fiber: 9.7g, Total Fat: 6.5g, Total Carbs: 82.5g, Protein: 4.4g.

Choco-Chunk Banana Ice Cream with Choco-Fudge Ripple

Serve up your favorite frozen bananas rippled with exquisite chocolate for just the right amount of bad when it comes to healthy treat making. This recipe is definitely for the choc-o-holic at heart!

YIELD: 5-7 SERVINGS | PREP TIME: 5 MINUTES | COOK TIME: 5 MINUTES

INGREDIENTS:

16 frozen bananas, peeled
1 teaspoon vanilla extract
1/4 cup 85% dark chocolate, chopped
1/4 cup calorie free chocolate fudge

INSTRUCTIONS:

1. Place a large mixing bowl under the fruit chute and push the bananas through.
2. Add vanilla extract and dark chocolate chunks.
3. Mix until smooth.
4. Add soft serve in 1-inch layers to a rectangular airtight container. After first layer, drizzle fudge across the soft-serve. Add a second layer of soft-serve and repeat the drizzle until the container is full.
5. Scoop ice cream into individual bowls.
6. Freeze leftover soft-serve.

Nutritional Info: Calories: 308, Sodium: 34mg, Dietary Fiber: 7.3g, Total Fat: 3.8g, Total Carbs: 68.5g, Protein: 387.1g.

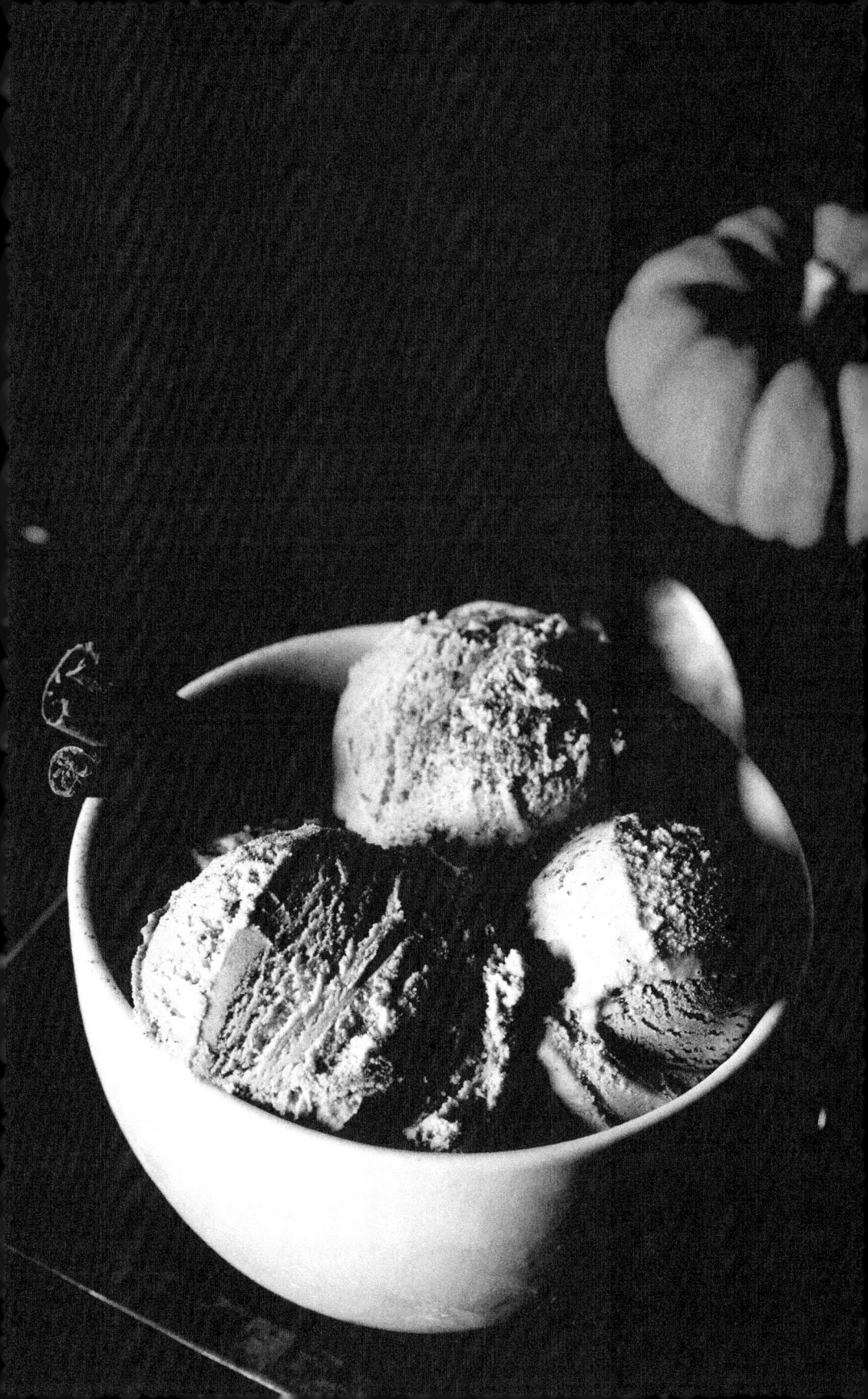

Pumpkin Cookie Ice Cream

Nothing says "sweet, spice and everything nice" like a bowl of this pumpkin cookie ice cream laced with decadence. Treat yourself or the whole family to a dessert that is savory, sweet and full of love.

YIELD: 4-6 SERVINGS | PREP TIME: 5 MINUTES | COOK TIME: 5 HOURS

INGREDIENTS:

- 12 frozen bananas, peeled
- 1 can pumpkin puree, frozen and sliced
- 3 tablespoons almond milk
- 1 teaspoon ground cinnamon
- 1 teaspoon allspice
- 1 teaspoon pure vanilla extract
- 1 teaspoon honey
- 1/2 cup gluten-free ginger snaps, chopped

INSTRUCTIONS:

1. Place a large mixing bowl under the fruit chute. Push the bananas and frozen pumpkin through.
2. Add almond milk, cinnamon, allspice, vanilla extract and honey to the bowl.
3. Stir until smooth and top with ginger snaps.
4. Place leftover soft-serve in an airtight container and freeze.

Nutritional Info: Calories: 332.3, Sodium: 88.3mg, Dietary Fiber: 8.1g, Total Fat: 5.1g, Total Carbs: 74.4g, Protein: 10.8g.

Chocolate Peanut Butter Banana Ice Cream

Perfectly sweet and packed with yummy peanut butter, this soft-serve is whipped with hunger fighting nut butter to keep you fuller longer—making this the perfect mid-day snack to keep you on your healthy diet.

YIELD: 3 SERVINGS | PREP TIME: 5 MINUTES | COOK TIME: 5 MINUTES

INGREDIENTS:

- 9 frozen bananas, peeled
- 2 tablespoons natural peanut butter, no sugar added
- 1/3 cup 85% dark cacao bar, chopped

INSTRUCTIONS:

1. Place a large mixing bowl under the fruit chute and push the bananas through.
2. Add peanut butter; mix until smooth.
3. Spoon into individual bowls and top with dark chocolate chunks.
4. Freeze leftovers in an airtight container.

Nutritional Info: Calories: 399, Sodium: 54mg, Dietary Fiber: 12.7g, Total Fat: 7.8g, Total Carbs: 88.2g, Protein: 8.3g.

Peanut Butter Frozen Banana

When you're in the mood for simple, this banana peanut butter ice cream is just what you should whip up. Treat the family to an after-school snack or simply curb cravings with this fiber-filled treat.

YIELD: 2-4 SERVINGS | PREP TIME: 5 MINUTES | COOK TIME: 5 MINUTES

INGREDIENTS:

- 9 frozen bananas, peeled
- 2 tablespoons natural peanut butter, no sugar added

INSTRUCTIONS:

1. Place a large mixing bowl under the fruit chute and push the bananas through.
2. Add the peanut butter and mix until smooth.
3. Serve in gluten-free waffle cones or scoop into individual bowls.

Nutritional Info: Calories: 283, Sodium: 39mg, Dietary Fiber: 7.4g, Total Fat: 4.9g, Total Carbs: 62.2g, Protein: 4.9g.

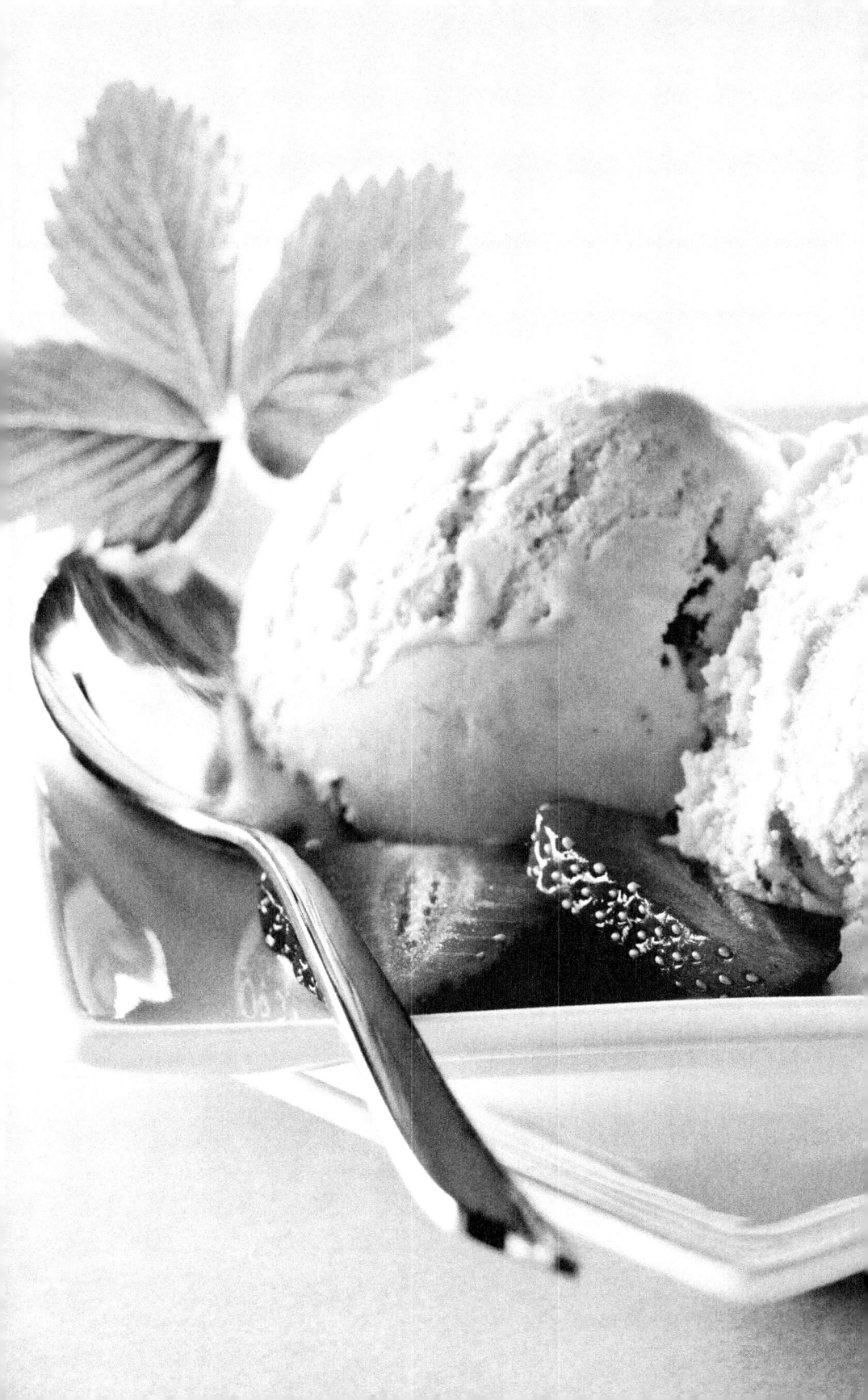

Strawberry Banana Ice Cream

Keep the weight off with yummy snacks that make you feel like you're truly indulging. This strawberry banana ice cream is just the treat to eat when you want something decadent that won't ruin your healthy habits.

YIELD: 2-4 SERVINGS | PREP TIME: 5 MINUTES | COOK TIME: 5 MINUTES

INGREDIENTS:

- 8 frozen bananas, peeled
- 1 cup frozen strawberries

INSTRUCTIONS:

1. Place a large mixing bowl under the fruit chute and push the bananas and strawberries through.
2. Stir until well-blended.
3. Serve in individual bowls.
4. Place leftover soft-serve in an airtight container and freeze.

Nutritional Info: Calories: 443, Sodium: 5mg, Dietary Fiber: 13.7g, Total Fat: 1.8g, Total Carbs: 113.3g, Protein: 5.6g.

Blueberry-Basil-Banana Soft-Serve

Whip up some super-yummy froyo right in the middle of your very own kitchen. Tangy blueberries and spicy basil make for some tantalizing dessert that will have your taste buds in heaven and your body full of super-food antioxidants.

YIELD: 4-6 SERVINGS | PREP TIME: 5 MINUTES | COOK TIME: 5 MINUTES

INGREDIENTS:

- 5 cups frozen blueberries
- 1 cup soy-based yogurt
- 1 tablespoon honey
- 1 teaspoon lemon juice
- 3 tablespoons fresh basil leaves, chopped

INSTRUCTIONS:

1. Place a large mixing bowl under the fruit chute and push the blueberries through.
2. Fold in soy-based yogurt, honey, lemon juice, and chopped basil.
3. Serve in individual bowls.
4. Place leftover soft-serve in an airtight container and freeze.

Nutritional Info: Calories: 109, Sodium: 14mg, Dietary Fiber: 2.9g, Total Fat: 1.2g, Total Carbs: 22.0g, Protein: 4.8g.

Pistachio Frozen Treat

Whisk your taste buds away to Saturday in the park with a taste of Italian summertime. Pistachio nut ice cream will remind you of creamy, intensely flavored gelato that is simply out of this world.

YIELD: 4 SERVINGS | PREP TIME: 5 MINUTES | COOK TIME: 5 MINUTES

INGREDIENTS:

- 12 frozen bananas, peeled
- 1-1/2 cups pistachio nuts, shelled
- 3 teaspoons brown sugar substitute
- 1/2 cup vanilla soy-based yogurt
- 1/2 teaspoon almond extract
- 3/4 cups pistachios, coarsely chopped

INSTRUCTIONS:

1. Process 1 and 1/2 cup pistachio nuts in a food processor until ground in a fine powder.
2. Place a large mixing bowl under the fruit chute and push the bananas through.
3. Fold in pistachio powder, brown sugar, yogurt, almond extract and mix until smooth.
4. Fold in chopped pistachios.
5. Serve in individual bowls and freeze leftover soft-serve in an airtight container.

Nutritional Info: Calories: 543, Sodium: 197mg, Dietary Fiber: 12.6g, Total Fat: 17.8g, Total Carbs: 946 g, Protein: 14.8g.

Date, Rum, & Pecan Ice Cream

Sometimes you just need a little boozy treat to wind down after a long day. This date, rum and pecan ice cream is just the dessert to quench your thirst. While it's not paleo, you can opt for rum flavoring to make it more paleo diet friendly.

YIELD: 2-4 SERVINGS | PREP TIME: 5 MINUTES | COOK TIME: 5 MINUTES

INGREDIENTS:

- 9 frozen bananas, peeled
- 12 frozen dates, pitted
- 1/2 cup vanilla soy-based yogurt
- 2 tablespoons sugar-free maple syrup
- 3 tablespoons cup spiced rum
- 1 cup pecans, toasted and coarsely chopped
- Pinch of pink Himalayan salt

INSTRUCTIONS:

1. Place a large mixing bowl under the fruit chute and push the bananas and dates through.
2. Mix in yogurt, maple syrup, salt and spiced rum until smooth.
3. Fold in chopped pecans.
4. Serve in individual bowls, and freeze leftover soft-serve in an airtight container.

Nutritional Info: Calories: 773, Sodium: 58mg, Dietary Fiber: 9.3g, Total Fat: 4.3g, Total Carbs: 88.2g, Protein: 8.0g.

Vanilla Avocado Banana Ice Cream

Packed with potassium and antioxidants, this scrumptious recipe is super-simple and absolutely delicious. The perfect snack for anyone looking to plump up their skin with some super-foods without packing on the pounds.

YIELD: 3 SERVINGS | PREP TIME: 5 MINUTES | COOK TIME: 5 MINUTES

INGREDIENTS:

- 9 frozen bananas, peeled
- 1 frozen avocado, peeled and pitted
- 1 tablespoon honey
- 1 teaspoon pure vanilla extract

INSTRUCTIONS:

1. Place a large mixing bowl under the fruit chute and push the bananas and avocado through.
2. Add honey and vanilla extract to the mixing bowl.
3. Mix until well-blended.
4. Serve in individual bowls and freeze leftovers in an airtight container.

Nutritional Info: Calories: 477, Sodium: 8mg, Dietary Fiber: 13.7g, Total Fat: 14.2g, Total Carbs: 92.6g, Protein: 5.1g.

Guinness-Milk Chocolate Ice Cream

Fold the creamy texture of Guinness into rich milk chocolate ice cream for one sincerely velvet dessert. This amazing dessert is best served with sugar-free shortbread cookies or as a decadent sundae topped with caramel sauce and toasted pecans.

YIELD: 4 SERVINGS | PREP TIME: 1 HOUR 5 MINUTES | COOK TIME: 5 MINUTES

INGREDIENTS:

- 12 frozen bananas, peeled
- 1 cup vanilla soy-based yogurt
- 3 tablespoons cocoa powder
- 1 tablespoon brown sugar substitute
- 1/3 cup Guinness Stout

INSTRUCTIONS:

1. Whip yogurt, cocoa powder and brown sugar substitute in a mixing bowl until smooth.
2. Refrigerate for 1 hour to set.
3. Place a large mixing bowl under the fruit chute and push the bananas through.
4. Fold in yogurt, then Guinness until smooth.
5. Serve in individual bowls and freeze leftover soft-serve in an airtight container.

Nutritional Info: Calories: 390, Sodium: 23mg, Dietary Fiber: 10.4g, Total Fat: 2.9g, Total Carbs: 88.6g, Protein: 10.4g.

Sweet Corn Ice Cream

An old-fashioned favorite, this luxurious ice cream is made from one of nature's simplest pleasures - sweet corn. With minimal ingredients, you might whip up this delicious frozen treat more than you imagine!
Try serving it in a gluten-free ice cream cone.

YIELD: 5-7 SERVINGS | PREP TIME: 5 MINUTES | COOK TIME: 5 MINUTES

INGREDIENTS:

- 2 bags of frozen corn
- 1 cup vanilla soy-based yogurt
- 1 tablespoon brown sugar-substitute

INSTRUCTIONS:

1. Place a large mixing bowl under the fruit chute and push the corn through.
2. Fold in yogurt and brown sugar substitute.
3. Serve in ice cream cones.
4. Freeze leftover soft-serve in an airtight container.

Nutritional Info: Calories: 50, Sodium: 11mg, Dietary Fiber: 0g, Total Fat: 0.8g, Total Carbs: 7.0g, Protein: 3.8g.

Almond-Banana Ice Cream

Almond butter and banana ice cream is definitely for the nut butter lover! Creamy, smooth this soft-serve hits the sweet spot in just the right scrumptious way.

YIELD: 4 SERVINGS | PREP TIME: 5 MINUTES | COOK TIME: 5 MINUTES

INGREDIENTS:

- 12 frozen bananas, peeled
- 1/2 cup almond butter
- 2 teaspoons pure vanilla extract
- 1 teaspoon honey

INSTRUCTIONS:

1. Place a large mixing bowl under the fruit chute and push the bananas through.
2. Mix in almond butter, vanilla extract and honey until well-blended.
3. Serve in individual servings.

Nutritional Info: Calories: 525, Sodium: 4mg, Dietary Fiber: 10.4g, Total Fat: 18.8g, Total Carbs: 88.1g, Protein: 10.5g.

S'mores Ice Cream Sandwiches

You don't need a campfire to whip up these nostalgic style treats! Nothing beats the crunch of graham cracker with marshmallow and chocolate - just this time it's a scrumptious ice cream sandwich!

YIELD: 4 SERVINGS | PREP TIME: 1 HOUR 5 MINUTES | COOK TIME: 5 MINUTES

INGREDIENTS:

- 6 frozen bananas
- 1 tablespoon coconut milk
- 1/2 cup vanilla soy-based yogurt
- 1/8 teaspoon cinnamon
- 1 tablespoons cocoa powder
- 1/4 cup ricemellow crème
- 4 graham crackers, broken into 8 square pieces

INSTRUCTIONS:

1. Whip yogurt, cocoa powder and cinnamon together and refrigerate for one hour.
2. Place a large mixing bowl under the fruit chute and push the bananas through.
3. Mix in yogurt mix until well-blended.
4. Drizzle in ricemellow and fold the ice cream to make a slight ripple.
5. Spoon onto graham crackers and top with a second graham cracker square.

Nutritional Info: Calories: 280, Sodium: 103.5mg, Dietary Fiber: 5.5g, Total Fat: 8.4g, Total Carbs: 58.4g, Protein: 7.4g.

Peach Ice Cream

Nothing quite hits the spot like an all too tempting bowl of peaches and cream. If you love the velvet texture of ice cream rippled with decadent peaches, you'll love this delicious soft-serve.

YIELD: 2-3 SERVINGS | PREP TIME: 5 MINUTES | COOK TIME: 5 MINUTES

INGREDIENTS:

- 3 cups frozen peaches
- 1 cup vanilla soy-based yogurt
- 1 tablespoon honey
- 1 cup frozen peaches, chopped

INSTRUCTIONS:

1. Place a large mixing bowl under the fruit chute and push the peaches through.
2. Mix in yogurt and honey until well-blended.
3. Fold in chopped peaches.
4. Spoon into individual bowls and freeze leftover soft-serve in an airtight container.

Nutritional Info: Calories: 168, Sodium: 25mg, Dietary Fiber: 3.4g, Total Fat: 2.1g, Total Carbs: 30.5g, Protein: 9.8g.

Concord Grape Sorbet

Nothing beats the juicy taste of a concord grape, and this fruit-filled sorbet is just the thing to keep your palate clean after dinner or in between tastings. Velvet, simple, and seductive, this sorbet is just a little on the heavenly side.

YIELD: 2-3 SERVINGS | PREP TIME: 3 MINUTES | COOK TIME: 5 MINUTES

INGREDIENTS:

4 cups frozen Concord grapes, stemmed

INSTRUCTIONS:

1. Place a large mixing bowl under the fruit chute and push the grapes through.
2. Spoon into individual bowls.
3. Freeze leftovers in an airtight container.

Nutritional Info: Calories: 62, Sodium: 2mg, Dietary Fiber: 0.8g, Total Fat: 0.3g, Total Carbs: 15.8g, Protein: 0.6g.

Salted Caramel Ice Cream

This French inspired soft-serve is as the French would say "c'est magnifique". A very magnificent treat that will take your taste buds on one fabulous taste adventure full of slightly salted, creamy caramel.

YIELD: 3 SERVINGS | PREP TIME: 3 MINUTES | COOK TIME: 5 MINUTES

INGREDIENTS:

- 1-1/4 cups coconut cream (heavy cream substitute)
- 1 cup brown sugar substitute
- 1/2 teaspoon pure vanilla extract
- 1/2 teaspoon fine ground sea salt
- 9 frozen bananas, peeled
- 1/2 cup vanilla soy-based yogurt

INSTRUCTIONS:

1. Heat a saucepan on medium heat. Pour brown sugar into the pan. Swirl the pan to heat sugar evenly until it starts to melt.
2. Fold in coconut cream when the sugar turns amber and stir until all of caramel dissolves.
3. Pour caramel into a mixing bowl and stir in sea salt and vanilla.
4. Set aside to cool to room temperature.
5. Place the mixing bowl with caramel under the fruit chute and push the bananas through.
6. Fold the yogurt into the soft-serve and mix until smooth.
7. Spoon into individual bowls.
8. Freeze leftovers in an airtight container.

Nutritional Info: Calories: 909, Sodium: 349mg, Dietary Fiber: 11.4g, Total Fat: 26.1g, Total Carbs: 152.7g, Protein: 11.7g.

Coconut-Rum Ice Cream

Vegans will rejoice in every single bite of this scrumptious ice cream! The perfect dessert for any vegan lifestyle, you'll never know this delicious ice cream doesn't have any dairy involved.

YIELD: 4 SERVINGS | PREP TIME: 5 MINUTES | COOK TIME: 5 MINUTES

INGREDIENTS:

12 frozen bananas, peeled
1 cup frozen coconut
2 tablespoons rum
3 tablespoons unsweetened coconut milk
1 teaspoon vanilla extract
1/3 cup raisins
1/3 cup shredded coconut

INSTRUCTIONS:

1. Place a large mixing bowl under the fruit chute and push the bananas and coconut through.
2. Mix in rum, coconut milk and vanilla extract until smooth.
3. Fold in raisins and shredded coconut.
4. Spoon into individual bowls.
5. Freeze leftovers in an airtight container.

Nutritional Info: Calories: 491, Sodium: 12mg, Dietary Fiber: 12.3g, Total Fat: 12.8g, Total Carbs: 95.2g, Protein: 5.4g.

Huckleberry Ice Cream

Huckleberry ice cream is the perfect mix of sweet and tart, blended into creamy ice cream for one uniquely delicious treat! Serve it up with fruit biscotti or gluten free wafers for a devilish dessert.

YIELD: 2-3 SERVINGS | PREP TIME: 5 MINUTES | COOK TIME: 5 MINUTES

INGREDIENTS:

- 2 cups frozen huckleberries
- 1 cup vanilla soy-based yogurt
- 1 tablespoon brown sugar-substitute

INSTRUCTIONS:

1. Place a large mixing bowl under the fruit chute and push the huckleberries through.
2. Fold in yogurt and brown sugar substitute.
3. Spoon into individual bowls and freeze leftover soft-serve in an airtight container.

Nutritional Info: Calories: 133, Sodium: 26mg, Dietary Fiber: 2.3g, Total Fat: 1.9g, Total Carbs: 21.1g, Protein: 8.5g.

Peanut Butter Ice Cream

If you love peanut butter and want to keep this ice cream vegan friendly, this delicious creamy treat is just the soft-serve to whip up. Smooth and velvety, serve this with banana chips and cacao chunks for one decadent dessert.

YIELD: 2-4 SERVINGS | PREP TIME: 5 MINUTES | COOK TIME: 5 MINUTES

INGREDIENTS:

- 9 frozen bananas, peeled
- 1 cup vanilla soy-based yogurt
- 3 tablespoons natural peanut butter, no sugar added

INSTRUCTIONS:

1. Place a large mixing bowl under the fruit chute and push the bananas through.
2. Add soy yogurt and peanut butter; mix until smooth.
3. Fold in raisins and shredded coconut.
4. Spoon into individual bowls.
5. Freeze leftovers in an airtight container.

Nutritional Info: Calories: 354, Sodium: 63mg, Dietary Fiber: 8.1g, Total Fat: 8.4g, Total Carbs: 69.2g, Protein: 8.4g.

Kaffir Lime Gelato

When it comes to whipping up an herbaceous filled creamy gelato, kaffir lime leaves are the perfect way to spice things up. This gorgeous, creamy treat is perfect after a spicy curry or alongside a glass of plum wine.

YIELD: 2-4 SERVINGS | PREP TIME: 5 MINUTES | COOK TIME: 5 MINUTES

INGREDIENTS:

- 9 frozen bananas, peeled
- 1 cup coconut cream
- 1 teaspoon lime juice
- 2 tablespoons lime zest
- 3 kaffir lime leaves, finely chopped

INSTRUCTIONS:

1. Place a large mixing bowl under the fruit chute and push the bananas through.
2. Fold in coconut cream, lime juice, and kaffir lime leaves.
3. Spoon into individual bowls and top with a sprinkle of lime zest.
4. Freeze leftovers in an airtight container.

Nutritional Info: Calories: 377, Sodium: 12mg, Dietary Fiber: 8.6g, Total Fat: 15.2g, Total Carbs: 65.0g, Protein: 4.3g.

PawPaw Ice Cream

Mix up a creamy treat with a tropical style fruit that is often referred to as one of the American Midwest's best kept secrets. With a musky sweet taste this ice cream might remind you of creamy bananas mixed with smooth mango.

YIELD: 3 SERVINGS | PREP TIME: 5 MINUTES | COOK TIME: 5 MINUTES

INGREDIENTS:

- 9 frozen paw paws, peeled and seeded
- 1 cup coconut cream
- 3 tablespoons almond milk
- 1 teaspoon pure vanilla extract
- 2 tablespoons honey

INSTRUCTIONS:

1. Place a large mixing bowl under the fruit chute and push the paw paws through.
2. Fold in coconut cream, almond milk, vanilla and honey.
3. Spoon into individual bowls and freeze leftovers in an airtight container.

Nutritional Info: Calories: 669, Sodium: 93mg, Dietary Fiber: 18.4g, Total Fat: 25.3g, Total Carbs: 119.2g, Protein: 6.8g.

Banana Ice Cream with Walnut Chip

The banana bread lover in you that wants to stay away from gluten will absolutely fall in love with this creamy delectable treat. Easy to make, you'll want to keep a gallon of this in the freezer for a healthy brunch treat to serve with gluten free vanilla wafers.

YIELD: 5 SERVINGS | PREP TIME: 5 MINUTES | COOK TIME: 5 MINUTES

INGREDIENTS:

- 15 bananas, sliced and frozen
- 1 tablespoon honey
- 1/2 teaspoon cinnamon
- 1/4 cup walnuts, chopped
- 1/2 cup 85% dark cacao bar, chopped

INSTRUCTIONS:

1. Place a large mixing bowl under the fruit chute and push the bananas through.
2. Mix in honey, cinnamon, walnuts, and dark chocolate chunks until well-blended.
3. Spoon into individual bowls.
4. Freeze leftovers in an airtight container.

Nutritional Info: Calories: 386, Sodium: 5mg, Dietary Fiber: 12.3g, Total Fat: 6.0g, Total Carbs: 89.8g, Protein: 6.9g.

Banana-Raisin Froyo

Take a step back to your childhood with a creamy mix of soft-serve blended with the delicious taste of Ants on a Log. A scrumptious treat for all ages, this one will be super popular with the kids just because of its cool name alone.

YIELD: 3 SERVINGS | PREP TIME: 5 MINUTES | COOK TIME: 5 MINUTES

INGREDIENTS:

- 9 frozen bananas, peeled
- 3 tablespoons natural peanut butter, no sugar added
- 1/3 cup raisins, yogurt covered raisins or chocolate covered raisins

INSTRUCTIONS:

1. Place a large mixing bowl under the fruit chute and push the bananas through.
2. Mix in peanut butter until well-blended.
3. Spoon into individual bowls and top with your favorite raisins.
4. Freeze leftovers in an airtight container.

Nutritional Info: Calories: 457, Sodium: 79mg, Dietary Fiber: 10.7g, Total Fat: 9.3g, Total Carbs: 96.8g, Protein: 8.3g.

Blueberry Banana Ice Cream

Blend up some super-food antioxidants for healthy skin and a healthy dose of muscle and joint lubricating potassium for one sweet treat full of health benefits. Your healthy lifestyle will love this soft-serve treat all day long!

YIELD: 3-5 SERVINGS | PREP TIME: 5 MINUTES | COOK TIME: 5 MINUTES

INGREDIENTS:

- 9 frozen bananas, peeled
- 1 cup frozen blueberries, stemmed
- 2 teaspoons pure vanilla extract

INSTRUCTIONS:

1. Place a large mixing bowl under the fruit chute and push the bananas and blueberries through.
2. Fold in vanilla extract and mix until well-blended.
3. Spoon into individual bowls, and freeze leftovers in an airtight container.

Nutritional Info: Calories: 210, Sodium: 2mg, Dietary Fiber: 6.2g, Total Fat: 0.8g, Total Carbs: 52.9g, Protein: 2.5g.

Banana Ice Cream with Cashew and Almond

Dress up your soft-serve with cashew and almonds for a boost of nutty vitamins and a pop of protein. A yummy soft-serve that is super-easy to whip up, you will love this for dessert or served on the side of a warm gluten-free brownie or slice of chocolate cake.

YIELD: 4 SERVINGS | PREP TIME: 5 MINUTES | COOK TIME: 5 MINUTES

INGREDIENTS:

- 9 frozen bananas, peeled
- 1/2 cup vanilla soy-based yogurt
- 1/4 cup cashews, chopped
- 1/4 cup almond slivers
- 1/4 cup banana chips, chopped

INSTRUCTIONS:

1. Place a large mixing bowl under the fruit chute and push the bananas through.
2. Fold in yogurt and mix until smooth.
3. Fold in cashews, almond and banana chips; mix well.
4. Serve in individual bowls and freeze leftovers in an airtight container.

Nutritional Info: Calories: 372, Sodium: 23mg, Dietary Fiber: 8.1g, Total Fat: 9.0g, Total Carbs: 69.2g, Protein: 11.3g.

Neapolitan Banana Ice Cream

For those days when you just can't decide whether you love vanilla, chocolate or strawberry ice cream—why not have all three? This delicious recipe is super-scrumptious alongside a piece of gluten-free birthday cake or classically served on its own.

YIELD: 4 SERVINGS | PREP TIME: 5 MINUTES | COOK TIME: 30 MINUTES

INGREDIENTS:

- 12 frozen bananas, peeled
- 2 cups frozen strawberries
- 1 tablespoon cocoa powder
- 1 cup vanilla soy-based yogurt

INSTRUCTIONS:

1. Mix 1/2 cup yogurt with cocoa powder and place in the refrigerator to set.
2. Place a mixing bowl under the fruit chute and push 6 bananas through.
3. Fold in 1/2 cup yogurt and mix until smooth; this is your vanilla ice cream.
4. Cover with cling wrap and place in the freezer until you mix up the other two soft-serve flavors.
5. Place a mixing bowl under the fruit chute and push 6 bananas through.
6. Fold in the chocolate yogurt and mix until smooth.
7. Cover with cling film and set aside in the freezer while you mix up the strawberry soft-serve.
8. Place a mixing bowl under the fruit chute and push the strawberries through.
9. Assemble the Neapolitan banana ice cream by scraping the vanilla ice cream into one side of an 8-by-5-inch loaf pan. Using an icing spatula, push the vanilla so it is flush and forms a wall.
10. Fill the middle third of the pan by adding the chocolate ice cream. Use an icing spatula to form a wall.
11. Fill the last third of the pan with strawberry-banana ice cream.
12. Scoop down the pan to make scoops of all three flavors.
13. Serve in single serving bowls and freeze leftovers.

Nutritional Info: Calories: 385, Sodium: 23mg, Dietary Fiber: 11.0g, Total Fat: 2.7g, Total Carbs: 89.4g, Protein: 10.4g.

Pumpkin Soft-Serve with Candied Ginger and Dark Chocolate

Baby, it might be cold outside, but it doesn't mean you can't enjoy a bowl of creamy ice cream. This spiced, chocolate chunked treat is sure to tantalize your pumpkin loving taste buds.

YIELD: 4 SERVINGS | PREP TIME: 5 MINUTES | COOK TIME: 5 MINUTES

INGREDIENTS:

12 frozen bananas, peeled
1 cup coconut cream
3 tablespoons maple syrup
1/2 teaspoon cinnamon
1 teaspoon allspice
1 teaspoon pure vanilla extract
1/4 cup pumpkin puree
1/3 cup candied ginger, chopped
6 ounces 85% dark cacao bar, chopped

INSTRUCTIONS:

1. Place a large mixing bowl under the fruit chute and push the bananas through.
2. Add coconut cream, maple syrup, cinnamon, allspice, vanilla extract, and pumpkin puree to the mixing bowl and mix until smooth.
3. Fold in candied ginger and dark chocolate chunks and mix well.
4. Serve in individual bowls or waffle cones, and freeze leftovers in an airtight container.

Nutritional Info: Calories: 602, Sodium: 24mg, Dietary Fiber: 24.0g, Total Fat: 21.2g, Total Carbs: 120.4g, Protein: 13.2g.

Almond Torte Mascarpone Ice Cream

Almond Torte Mascarpone Ice Cream literally is like a little slice of heaven. A bowl of this creamy almond filled soft-serve is almost like eating a slice of America's Best Cake from Prantl's Bakery right out of Pittsburgh. Absolutely scrumptious!

YIELD: 2-4 SERVINGS | PREP TIME: 5 MINUTES | COOK TIME: 5 MINUTES

INGREDIENTS:

- 9 frozen bananas, peeled
- 1/2 cup coconut cream, chilled
- 1/2 cup vanilla soy-based yogurt
- 1/2 teaspoon honey
- 2 teaspoons almond extract
- 1/4 cup soy-based vegan mascarpone
- 1/4 cup almond torte cake, cut into pieces
- 1/4 cup almonds, sliced

INSTRUCTIONS:

1. Place a large mixing bowl under the fruit chute and push the bananas through.
2. Add coconut cream, yogurt, honey, almond extract and mascarpone cheese and mix until smooth.
3. Fold in almond torte cake and mix lightly.
4. Scoop into ice cream cones and top with almond slices.
5. Freeze leftovers in an airtight container.

Nutritional Info: Calories: 445, Sodium: 63mg, Dietary Fiber: 8.3g, Total Fat: 15.2g, Total Carbs: 71.5g, Protein: 12.6g.

Rum and Raisin Ice Cream

There really is something special about the burnt vanilla spiced taste of rum mixed with the sun picked sweet of a raisin. Mix these two flavors with cream soft-serve and you've got one dastardly devilish dessert.

YIELD: 3-5 SERVINGS | PREP TIME: 24 HOURS 5 MINUTES | COOK TIME: 5 MINUTES

INGREDIENTS:

- 12 frozen bananas, peeled
- 1/2 cup coconut cream, chilled
- 1 teaspoon pure vanilla extract
- 3 tablespoons brown sugar substitute
- 1/2 cup raisins
- 1/2 cup spiced rum

INSTRUCTIONS:

1. Soak the raisins in the spiced rum overnight.
2. Place a large mixing bowl under the fruit chute and push the bananas through.
3. Add coconut cream, vanilla extract, brown sugar and 1 teaspoon of rum from the raisins; mix until well-blended.
4. Drain the raisins and fold them into the soft-serve.
5. Scoop into individual bowls.
6. Freeze leftovers in an airtight container.

Nutritional Info: Calories: 440, Sodium: 8mg, Dietary Fiber: 8.4g, Total Fat: 6.7g, Total Carbs: 84.8g, Protein: 4.1g.

Homemade Coco-Mango Sorbet

Coconut mango ice cream is a little taste of Asia in a bowl. Perfectly blended for a sweet creamy soft-serve that is sure to make your taste buds explode. Enjoy this soft-serve on top of a ball of coconut sticky rice for a truly Asian experience.

YIELD: 3 SERVINGS | PREP TIME: 5 MINUTES | COOK TIME: 5 MINUTES

INGREDIENTS:

- 3 frozen mangoes, chopped
- 3 tablespoons unsweetened coconut milk
- 1/2 cup coconut cream, chilled
- 1 teaspoon pure vanilla extract
- 1 teaspoon honey
- 1/4 cup unsweetened coconut, shredded

INSTRUCTIONS:

1. Place a large mixing bowl under the fruit chute and push the mangos through.
2. Add coconut milk, coconut cream, vanilla extract and honey; mix until well-blended.
3. Scoop into individual bowls and top with shredded coconut.
4. Freeze leftovers in an airtight container.

Nutritional Info: Calories: 231, Sodium: 12mg, Dietary Fiber: 3.6g, Total Fat: 15.6g, Total Carbs: 23.2g, Protein: 2.0g.

Citrus-Mint Sorbet

Blend tropical fruits for a fun, fruity treat and spike it with refreshing mint for a unique take on tropical style froyo. This cool treat is absolutely delicious on hot sunny days to cool off in absolute fresh style.

YIELD: 5 SERVINGS | PREP TIME: 5 MINUTES | COOK TIME: 5 MINUTES

INGREDIENTS:

- 3 frozen bananas
- 6 frozen lemons, peeled and seeded
- 3 frozen oranges, peeled and seeded
- 1 cup plain soy-based yogurt
- 1 tablespoon honey
- 2 tablespoons fresh mint, chopped

INSTRUCTIONS:

1. Place a large mixing bowl under the fruit chute and push the bananas, lemons and oranges through.
2. Mix in yogurt and honey until well-blended.
3. Fold in chopped mint.
4. Spoon into individual bowls and freeze leftover soft-serve in an airtight container.

Nutritional Info: Calories: 184, Sodium: 18mg, Dietary Fiber: 6.6g, Total Fat: 1.5g, Total Carbs: 41.1g, Protein: 7.3g.

Blueberry Frozen Soy Yogurt

When it comes to vegan treats that are paleo diet friendly and lactose free, you don't have to skimp on the rich ingredients in order to whip up something delicious and tasty!

YIELD: 2-4 SERVINGS | PREP TIME: 5 MINUTES | COOK TIME: 5 MINUTES

INGREDIENTS:

- 5 cups frozen blueberries, stemmed
- 2-3/4 cups unsweetened plain soy yogurt
- 3 tablespoons blueberry jam

INSTRUCTIONS:

1. Place a large mixing bowl under the fruit chute and push the blueberries through.
2. Fold yogurt and jam into the bowl.
3. Mix until smooth.
4. Spoon into individual bowls.
5. Freeze leftovers in an airtight container.

Nutritional Info: Calories: 272, Sodium: 15mg, Dietary Fiber: 5.8g, Total Fat: 4.8g, Total Carbs: 53.2g, Protein: 8.3g.

Cherry-Coconut Ice Cream Sandwiches

A twist on the traditional ice cream sandwich, this creamy cherry filled dessert will still hit a sinful spot. If you love shortbread cookies, cherries and everything nice this soft-serve is the perfect dessert.

YIELD: 4 SERVINGS | PREP TIME: 5 MINUTES | COOK TIME: 5 MINUTES

INGREDIENTS:

- 5 cups frozen cherries, pitted
- 1/4 cup coconut cream, chilled
- 1 teaspoon pure vanilla extract
- 1 teaspoon honey
- 6 shortbread cookies, gluten-free or sugar free
- 1/4 cup unsweetened coconut, shredded

INSTRUCTIONS:

1. Place a large mixing bowl under the fruit chute and push the cherries through.
2. Fold in coconut cream, vanilla extract and honey and mix until well-blended.
3. Pour shredded coconut onto a piece of parchment paper.
4. Assemble the sandwiches by scooping one scoop of soft-serve onto a cookie. Place a second cookie on top of the scoop.
5. Hold the sandwich in between your hands and roll the ice cream side in the shredded coconut.
6. Freeze any leftovers in an airtight container.

Nutritional Info: Calories: 186, Sodium: 489mg, Dietary Fiber: 2.3g, Total Fat: 5.3g, Total Carbs: 32.9g, Protein: 0.8g.

Malted Milk Ice Cream Bonbons

A sinfully sweet treat, malted milk ice cream bonbons are super-easy to whip up. Enjoy these delicious little ice cream treats with your favorite glass of red wine or as an after-dinner aperitif with a smooth glass of scotch.

YIELD: 5-7 SERVINGS | PREP TIME: 15 MINUTES | COOK TIME: 25 MINUTES

INGREDIENTS:

- 6 frozen bananas, peeled
- 1 cup chocolate covered malted milk balls
- 1 cup malted milk powder

INSTRUCTIONS:

1. Crush the malted milk balls in a plastic bag with a meat tenderizer or food process for a few minutes.
2. Pour malted milk ball pieces into a bowl.
3. Pour malted milk powder into a second bowl.
4. Place a mixing bowl under the fruit chute and push the bananas through.
5. Scoop out 1 tablespoon of banana soft-serve. Roll it into a ball.
6. Roll the ball in malted milk powder, then roll it in the malted milk ball pieces.
7. Place ice cream bonbon on a separate plate.
8. Repeat until all bonbons are rolled
9. Freeze bonbons for 20 minutes and enjoy!

Nutritional Info: Calories: 176, Sodium: 116mg, Dietary Fiber: 2.6g, Total Fat: 1.0g, Total Carbs: 34.7g, Protein: 9.1g.

Cookie Dough Ice Cream

Put a little love in your healthy lifestyle with some super-yummy, decadent vegan cookie dough ice cream. This ice cream is also one very sweet treat for anyone ready to go on a little detox diet. Feed your sweet tooth something extraordinary when you whip up your very own healthy version of cookie dough ice cream.

YIELD: 2 SERVINGS | PREP TIME: 1 HOUR 15 MINUTES | COOK TIME: 5 MINUTES

INGREDIENTS:

- 6 frozen bananas, peeled
- 1/2 cup almonds
- 3 soft dates, pitted
- 1/4 teaspoon pure vanilla extract
- Pinch of pink Himalayan salt
- 1 tablespoon 85% dark cacao bar, chopped into fine chunks or slivers

INSTRUCTIONS:

1. Pulse the walnuts in a small food processor until finely ground. Add the dates, vanilla, and Himalayan salt. Pulse again until the ingredients form a sticky dough.
2. Transfer the dough to a small mixing bowl.
3. Fold in dark chocolate chunks.
4. Line a baking sheet with parchment paper.
5. Roll the dough into 1/4 inch balls and freeze to set for 1 hour.
6. Place a mixing bowl under the fruit chute and push the bananas through.
7. Fold the cookie dough into the soft-serve.
8. Serve in individual bowls and freeze any leftovers.

Nutritional Info: Calories: 495, Sodium: 82mg, Dietary Fiber: 14.0g, Total Fat: 13.5g, Total Carbs: 96.8g, Protein: 9.7g.

Lemon Buttermilk Pie Ice Cream

Pie lovers rejoice! Lemon buttermilk pie ice cream tastes just like a slice of heaven. Serve this delicious pie like creamy treat up in a waffle cone or in a bowl topped with crushed gluten-free pie crust for a guilt free dessert.

YIELD: 3-5 SERVINGS | PREP TIME: 5 MINUTES | COOK TIME: 5 MINUTES

INGREDIENTS:

- 9 frozen bananas, peeled
- 1/2 cup unsweetened almond milk
- 1/4 cup vanilla soy-based yogurt
- 3 teaspoons brown sugar substitute
- 3 tablespoons lemon juice
- 1 teaspoon lemon zest
- 1/2 cup frozen pie crust bits

INSTRUCTIONS:

1. Place a mixing bowl under the fruit chute and push the bananas through.
2. Fold the almond milk, coconut cream, brown sugar, lemon juice, yogurt and lemon zest into the soft-serve.
3. Mix until well-blended.
4. Scoop into a cone or bowl and top with crushed pie pieces.
5. Freeze leftovers in an airtight container.

Nutritional Info: Calories: 285.4, Sodium: 70.4mg, Dietary Fiber: 5.7g, Total Fat: 3.88g, Total Carbs: 58.4g, Protein: 20.1g.

Vegan Coconut Raspberry Ice Cream

Sometimes you simply crave creamy ice cream mixed with scrumptious raspberries. If you're Vegan, you're in for a treat. If you're not, you're still in for a delicious treat because you'll simply never know the difference when you make this soft-serve.

YIELD: 2-4 SERVINGS | PREP TIME: 5 MINUTES | COOK TIME: 5 MINUTES

INGREDIENTS:

- 9 frozen bananas, peeled
- 1 cup frozen raspberries
- 3 tablespoons unsweetened coconut milk
- 1/2 teaspoon sugar substitute
- 1 teaspoon pure vanilla extract

INSTRUCTIONS:

1. Place a large mixing bowl under the fruit chute and push the bananas and raspberries through.
2. Add the coconut milk, sugar substitute and vanilla extract.
3. Mix until well-blended.
4. Serve in singles servings and freeze any leftovers.

Nutritional Info: Calories: 283, Sodium: 5mg, Dietary Fiber: 9.2g, Total Fat: 3.8g, Total Carbs: 65.6g, Protein: 3.5g.

Coconut Cake Frosting Ice Cream

Topped with naturally sweet coconut, this delicious, simple recipe is sinfully sweet and out of this world. Serve your coconut cake frosting ice cream alongside a piece of gluten-free yellow cake or topped with gluten-free animal crackers.

YIELD: 2-3 SERVINGS | PREP TIME: 5 MINUTES | COOK TIME: 5 MINUTES

INGREDIENTS:

- 2 cups frozen coconut chunks (meat)
- 1 cup coconut cream, chilled
- 2 tablespoons sugar substitute
- 1 teaspoon pure vanilla extract
- 1/2 cup unsweetened coconut, shredded

INSTRUCTIONS:

1. Place a mixing bowl under the fruit chute.
2. Push the coconut meat through.
3. Add the coconut cream, sugar and vanilla extract.
4. Mix until well-blended.
5. Serve individual bowls and top with shredded coconut.
6. Freeze leftovers in an airtight container.

Nutritional Info: Calories: 464, Sodium: 25mg, Dietary Fiber: 7.8g, Total Fat: 41.3g, Total Carbs: 22.8g, Protein: 4.1g.

Lemon-Aid Sorbet

Some sorbets dare to be different just like a bowl of Arnold Palmer inspired half tea, half lemonade. Perfect on any hot summer day or as a refreshing snack after you hit the golf course.

YIELD: 2-4 SERVINGS | PREP TIME: 5 MINUTES | COOK TIME: 24 HOURS 20 MINUTES

INGREDIENTS:

- 2 cups water
- 4 black or orange pekoe tea bags
- 3 frozen bananas, peeled
- 1/4 cup lemon juice
- 1 tablespoon bourbon
- 1 teaspoon honey

INSTRUCTIONS:

1. Bring two cups of water to a boil on high heat in a medium saucepan.
2. Add tea bags and remove from heat.
3. Steep tea for 15 to 20 minutes.
4. Pour tea into two ice cube trays and freeze overnight.
5. Place a mixing bowl under the fruit chute and push the bananas and tea ice cubes through.
6. Add lemon juice, bourbon, and honey to the mixing bowl.
7. Blend until smooth.
8. Spoon into individual bowls and freeze leftover soft-serve in an airtight container.

Nutritional Info: Calories: 96, Sodium: 8mg, Dietary Fiber: 2.4g, Total Fat: 0.4g, Total Carbs: 23.0g, Protein: 1.1g.

Maple Bacon Ice Cream

Combine the smoky taste of bourbon with sweet maple. Blend it with creamy ice cream and top it with candied bacon for the perfect savory sweet treat that is absolutely to die for!

YIELD: 2-4 SERVINGS | PREP TIME: 5 MINUTES | COOK TIME: 30 MINUTES

INGREDIENTS:

- 9 frozen bananas, peeled
- 1/2 cup vanilla soy-based yogurt
- 3 strips turkey bacon, maple flavored, cooked and chopped
- 1 cup brown sugar substitute
- 2 tablespoons bourbon
- 1 teaspoon maple syrup

INSTRUCTIONS:

1. Heat a medium saucepan on medium heat and add the brown sugar.
2. Swirl the pan to keep the sugar from burning; melt until dark amber.
3. Fold in the chopped turkey bacon.
4. Place candied turkey bacon onto a wax paper line baking sheet to cool.
5. Place a mixing bowl under the fruit chute and push the bananas through.
6. Add yogurt, bourbon and maple syrup to the mixing bowl.
7. Blend until smooth.
8. Fold candied bacon into the soft-serve.
9. Spoon into individual bowls and freeze leftover soft-serve in an airtight container.

Nutritional Info: Calories: 556, Sodium: 115mg, Dietary Fiber: 6.9g, Total Fat: 2.4g, Total Carbs: 112.1g, Protein: 11.0g.

Chiquita Banana Ice Cream

If you love Chiquita bananas, you'll dance to the rhythm of every bite of this creamy soft-serve treat. Simple, delicious and "oh, so very healthy"—this frozen treat can be served up in just minutes for delicious fun.

YIELD: 3-5 SERVINGS | PREP TIME: 5 MINUTES | COOK TIME: 5 MINUTES

INGREDIENTS:

- 9 frozen bananas, peeled
- 1 cup coconut cream
- 2 teaspoons lime juice
- 2 teaspoons honey
- 2 teaspoons pure vanilla extract

INSTRUCTIONS:

1. Place a large mixing bowl under the fruit chute and push the bananas through.
2. Fold in coconut cream, lime juice, honey and vanilla extract.
3. Mix until smooth.
4. Serve in individual bowls and freeze leftovers in an airtight container.

Nutritional Info: Calories: 317, Sodium: 10mg, Dietary Fiber: 6.7g, Total Fat: 12.1g, Total Carbs: 55.2g, Protein: 3.5g.

Passion Fruit Ice Cream

Whip up your passion of delicious fruit in this scrumptious, simple recipe. The best part about this recipe is that if ripe passion fruit isn't readily available—you can still feed your soul with one super easy substitute.

YIELD: 2-4 SERVINGS | PREP TIME: 5 MINUTES | COOK TIME: 5 MINUTES

INGREDIENTS:

 5 frozen passion fruit, peeled and seeded (alternatively use 2 cans of frozen passion fruit juice sliced and halved)
 1/2 cup plain soy-based yogurt
 1 teaspoon of honey

INSTRUCTIONS:

1. Place a mixing bowl under the fruit chute and push the passion fruit or sliced juice through.
2. Add yogurt and honey.
3. Blend until smooth.
4. Spoon into individual bowls and freeze any leftovers.

Nutritional Info: Calories: 58, Sodium: 20mg, Dietary Fiber: 2.3g, Total Fat: 1.0g, Total Carbs: 8.4g, Protein: 4.7g.

Non-Dairy Peach Ice Cream

When it comes to whipping up one dreamy dairy-free dessert, it's so simple you might just make a whole gallon to freeze for endless peach ice cream. Perfect alongside peach cobbler, peach pie, peach dumplings or blended into a creamy milkshake—you will absolutely love this recipe if you love peaches.

YIELD: 3 SERVINGS | PREP TIME: 5 MINUTES | COOK TIME: 5 MINUTES

INGREDIENTS:

- 1 bag frozen peaches
- 1/2 cup vanilla soy-based yogurt
- 1 teaspoon honey

INSTRUCTIONS:

1. Place a mixing bowl under the fruit chute and push the peaches through.
2. Add yogurt and honey.
3. Mix until smooth.
4. Serve it up your favorite way.

Nutritional Info: Calories: 51, Sodium: 3mg, Dietary Fiber: 0.8g, Total Fat: 1.1g, Total Carbs: 9.2g, Protein: 2.0g.

Rosé Sherbet

Perfect for a New Year's Eve treat or the Sunday Brunch for ladies who lunch. Rosé Sorbet pairs perfectly with savory sweet potato hash and yogurt topped lemon lime polenta cake for one tantalizingly delicious meal. You'll definitely want to share this one with your friends.

YIELD: 3-5 SERVINGS | PREP TIME: 5 MINUTES | COOK TIME: 5 MINUTES

INGREDIENTS:

- 3 cups frozen raspberries
- 1/2 cup rosé wine
- Rose petals for garnish

INSTRUCTIONS:

1. Place a large mixing bowl under the fruit chute and push the raspberries through.
2. Add rosé wine and mix until well-blended
3. Scoop into champagne glasses and add a rose petal or two for garnish.

Nutritional Info: Calories: 58, Sodium: 2mg, Dietary Fiber: 4.8g, Total Fat: 0.5g, Total Carbs: 9.5g, Protein: 0.9g.

Banana Nutella Soft-Serve

Mix the creamy texture of banana soft-serve with the hazelnut chocolate decadence of Nutella and you've got one dreamy treat. Gelato is best served on a hot summer day while you take a break on the front porch or under the shade of a tree.

YIELD: 5-8 SERVINGS | PREP TIME: 5 MINUTES | COOK TIME: 5 MINUTES

INGREDIENTS:

- 16 frozen bananas, peeled
- 1 cup vanilla soy-based yogurt
- 1/3 cup Nutella

INSTRUCTIONS:

1. Place a mixing bowl under the fruit chute and push the bananas through.
2. Add yogurt and blend until smooth.
3. Spoon one inch of banana soft-serve into a loaf pan and smooth it over with an icing spatula.
4. Put Nutella in a plastic bag and cut one corner off.
5. Drizzle Nutella sporadically across the entire layer; Repeat until pan is full.
6. Serve in individual bowls and freeze leftover soft-serve in an airtight container.

Nutritional Info: Calories: 259, Sodium: 7mg, Dietary Fiber: 6.6g, Total Fat: 2.9g, Total Carbs: 59.9g, Protein: 4.1g.

Fried Ice Cream

Whip up a delicious Mexican dessert right in the comfort of your own kitchen with this scrumptious Mexican fried ice cream. Drizzle it with chocolate, top it with whip cream, and savor this soft-serve on a day when comfort food is just what your soul calls for!

YIELD: 4 SERVINGS | PREP TIME: 5 MINUTES | COOK TIME: 15 MINUTES

INGREDIENTS:

- 2 cups cornflakes, crushed
- 1/4 cup unsalted butter
- 12 frozen bananas, peeled
- 1/2 cup vanilla soy-based yogurt
- 1/2 teaspoon cinnamon
- Chocolate sauce (for topping)
- Truwhip (for topping)

INSTRUCTIONS:

1. Melt butter in a saucepan on medium heat.
2. Add crushed cornflakes and cook until golden brown.
3. Pour the cornflake mix into a shallow bowl and set aside.
4. Place a mixing bowl under the fruit chute and push the bananas through.
5. Add yogurt and cinnamon to the mixing bowl and blend until smooth.
6. Use an ice cream scoop to scoop out one serving.
7. Roll it in the cornflake mix.
8. Place the cornflake rolled scoop into a bowl and top with chocolate sauce and Truwhip; repeat for additional servings.
9. Freeze leftover soft-serve in an airtight container.

Nutritional Info: Calories: 499, Sodium: 199mg, Dietary Fiber: 9.8g, Total Fat: 13.5g, Total Carbs: 94.8g, Protein: 9.2g.

Root Beer Barrel Ice Cream

Fans of sarsaparilla, birch beer or sassafras will no doubt love this creamy root beer flavored treat. Blend the creamy flavor of ice cream and root beer for a dreamy treat that will make your senses soar. Enjoy Root Beer Barrel ice cream with Italian wafers for a malt shoppe style treat.

YIELD: 3-5 SERVINGS | PREP TIME: 5 MINUTES | COOK TIME: 5 MINUTES

INGREDIENTS:

- 10 frozen bananas, peeled
- 1 cup vanilla soy-based yogurt
- 2 teaspoons honey
- 1-1/2 teaspoons root beer extract, frozen
- 5 root beer barrel candies, crushed

INSTRUCTIONS:

1. Place a mixing bowl under the fruit chute and push the bananas through.
2. Add yogurt, honey and root beer extract to the mixing bowl, and blend until smooth.
3. Fold in crushed root beer barrels.
4. Spoon into individual bowls and freeze leftover soft-serve in an airtight container.

Nutritional Info: Calories: 337.6, Sodium: 22.2mg, Dietary Fiber: 7.7g, Total Fat: 2.1g, Total Carbs: 77.3g, Protein: 9.0g.

Chocolate Decadence Ice Cream

When you think decadent, chocolate definitely comes to mind. What makes this yummy treat so decadent is the fact that it's topped with rich chocolate granola and chocolate sauce. For the chocolate lover at heart this one packs one very rich punch!

YIELD: 2-4 SERVINGS | PREP TIME: 5 MINUTES | COOK TIME: 5 MINUTES

INGREDIENTS:

- 9 frozen bananas, peeled
- 1/2 cup vanilla soy-based yogurt
- 1/4 cup cream of coconut, chilled
- 1 teaspoon honey
- 1 cup chocolate granola
- 1/2 cup chocolate sauce
- 3 tablespoons 85% dark cacao bar, chopped

INSTRUCTIONS:

1. Place a mixing bowl under the fruit chute and push the bananas through.
2. Add yogurt, cream of coconut and honey to the mixing bowl.
3. Blend until smooth.
4. Fold in a 1/2 cup chocolate granola.
5. Spoon into individual bowls.
6. Top each bowl with chocolate sauce, dark chocolate chunks and additional granola.

Nutritional Info: Calories: 461, Sodium: 41mg, Dietary Fiber: 14.0g, Total Fat: 27.11g, Total Carbs: 102.9g, Protein: 20.3g.

Oat & Dulce de Leche Sorbet

Indulge your senses in the creamy texture of dulce de leche. With fiber packed oats in the mix, this sweet treat will keep you fuller longer. Perfect for mid-morning snack or as an after dinner treat to curb hunger before bedtime.

YIELD: 4-6 SERVINGS | PREP TIME: 5 MINUTES | COOK TIME: 5 MINUTES

INGREDIENTS:

- 9 frozen bananas, peeled
- 1/2 cup vanilla soy-based yogurt
- 1 teaspoon honey
- 1 teaspoon spiced rum, frozen
- 1 cup honey toasted granola
- 1/2 cup dulce de leche

INSTRUCTIONS:

1. Place a mixing bowl under the fruit chute and push the bananas through.
2. Add yogurt, honey, and spiced rum to the mixing bowl.
3. Blend until smooth.
4. Fold in the honey toasted granola.
5. Spoon into individual bowls, and drizzle with dulce de leche.

Nutritional Info: Calories: 304, Sodium: 51mg, Dietary Fiber: 8.3g, Total Fat: 11.9g, Total Carbs: 79.5g, Protein: 12.1g.

Orange Ice Cream with Dark Chocolate Chip

If you love chocolate orange candy, you will adore this velvety smooth soft-serve. Trade your chocolate orange for a healthy bowl of orange dark chocolate chip ice cream. Enjoy it on its own or in the delicious, flakey crunch of a gluten-free ice cream cone.

YIELD: 3-5 SERVINGS | PREP TIME: 1 HOUR 5 MINUTES | COOK TIME: 5 MINUTES

INGREDIENTS:

- 9 frozen bananas, peeled
- 1 cup frozen oranges, peeled and seeded
- 1/2 cup vanilla soy-based yogurt
- 3 teaspoons cocoa powder
- 3 tablespoons 85% dark cacao bar, chopped

INSTRUCTIONS:

1. Mix the cocoa powder into the Greek yogurt and chill in the refrigerator for 1 hour.
2. Place a mixing bowl under the fruit chute.
3. Push the bananas and oranges through.
4. Add the chocolate yogurt and mix until well-blended.
5. Fold in the dark chocolate chunks.
6. Scoop into a cone or bowl.
7. Freeze leftovers in an airtight container.

Nutritional Info: Calories: 265.6, Sodium: 17mg, Dietary Fiber: 7.2g, Total Fat: 3.6g, Total Carbs: 56.5g, Protein: 7.9g.

Peach Ice Cream

Life tastes so much sweeter with delectable desserts like this peach cobbler ice cream. Simple, sweet, and just the right amount of love and you will have one decadent dish the whole family will thank you for!

YIELD: 4-6 SERVINGS | PREP TIME: 5 MINUTES | COOK TIME: 5 MINUTES

INGREDIENTS:

- 1/2 cup oats
- 1/2 cup pecans, chopped
- 1/4 cup brown sugar substitute
- 1/4 cup margarine, unsalted
- 1 teaspoon cinnamon
- 2 bags of frozen peaches
- 1/2 cup vanilla soy-based yogurt
- 1 teaspoon honey

INSTRUCTIONS:

1. Heat a medium saucepan on medium heat.
2. Add margarine and brown sugar.
3. Once melted, fold in oats, chopped pecans, and cinnamon.
4. Remove from heat and lay out on a parchment lined baking sheet to cool.
5. Place a mixing bowl under the fruit chute and push the peaches through.
6. Add yogurt and honey to the mixing bowl, and blend until smooth.
7. Spoon into individual bowls, and top with cinnamon toasted oat mix.

Nutritional Info: Calories: 208, Sodium: 64mg, Dietary Fiber: 2.4g, Total Fat: 10.5g, Total Carbs: 23.3g, Protein: 4.8g.

Tahini and Lemon Curd Ice Cream

Mix the warm essence of tahini with the refreshing taste of lemon curd for one seriously cool dessert. While you'll be basking in the freshness of this seedy little soft-serve, you'll also be raking in the health benefits. Tahini is well-known for its amazing potential to lower cholesterol and fight heart disease.

YIELD: 4 SERVINGS | PREP TIME: 5 MINUTES | COOK TIME: 5 MINUTES

INGREDIENTS:

- 12 frozen bananas, peeled
- 1/2 cup tahini paste
- 2 teaspoons pure vanilla extract
- 3 tablespoons lemon curd
- 1 teaspoon honey

INSTRUCTIONS:

1. Place a mixing bowl under the fruit chute and push the bananas through.
2. Add tahini, vanilla extract, lemon curd and honey to the mixing bowl.
3. Blend until smooth.
4. Spoon into individual bowls and freeze leftover soft-serve in an airtight container.

Nutritional Info: Calories: 538, Sodium: 38mg, Dietary Fiber: 12.0g, Total Fat: 17.75g, Total Carbs: 95.8g, Protein: 9.0g.

Chocolate Malted Whopper Ice Cream

Mix up a killer bowl of movie theatre treat inspired ice cream with this delicious chocolate malted Whopper ice cream! Nothing beats ice cream blended with your favorite candies and if you like malted milk balls covered in chocolate this soft-serve is sinfully sweet.

YIELD: 3-5 SERVINGS | PREP TIME: 5 MINUTES | COOK TIME: 5 MINUTES

INGREDIENTS:

- 10 frozen bananas, peeled
- 1 cup coconut cream, chilled
- 1 tablespoon honey
- 1 teaspoon vanilla
- 1/2 cup Whoppers or chocolate covered malted milk balls

INSTRUCTIONS:

1. Place a mixing bowl under the fruit chute and push the bananas through.
2. Add coconut cream, honey and vanilla extract to the mixing bowl.
3. Blend until smooth.
4. Fold in whoppers, and spoon into individual servings.

Nutritional Info: Calories: 448.8, Sodium: 69.4mg, Dietary Fiber: 7.2g, Total Fat: 18.9g, Total Carbs: 67.9g, Protein: 8.6g

Banana Sorbet with Rose and Pistachio

If you love pistachios and herbaceous delights, one delicious bowl of Syrian ice will hit the spot. A little something sweet, a little something you can't quite put your finger on and whole lotta love go into this surprisingly scrumptious soft-serve.

YIELD: 2-4 SERVINGS | PREP TIME: 5 MINUTES | COOK TIME: 5 MINUTES

INGREDIENTS:

- 6 frozen bananas, peeled
- 1/4 cup vanilla soy-based yogurt
- 1 tablespoon honey
- 1/2 teaspoon rose water
- 1/2 cup pistachios, chopped

INSTRUCTIONS:

1. Place a mixing bowl under the fruit chute and push the bananas through.
2. Add yogurt, honey and rose water to the mixing bowl.
3. Blend until smooth.
4. Spoon into individual bowls, and top each serving with a generous portion of chopped pistachios.
5. Freeze leftover soft-serve in an airtight container.

Nutritional Info: Calories: 224, Sodium: 47mg, Dietary Fiber: 5.4g, Total Fat: 4.4g, Total Carbs: 47.3g, Protein: 4.9g.

Cinnamon Cream Cheese Ice Cream

Think cinnamon cheesecake drizzled with homemade cinnamon syrup and that's exactly what you'll get when you whip up a batch of cinnamon cream cheese ice cream with cinnamon syrup. Talk about a taste bud explosion, this savory sweet treat is spiced just right.

YIELD: 4-5 SERVINGS | PREP TIME: 5 MINUTES | COOK TIME: 25 MINUTES

INGREDIENTS:

- 12 frozen bananas, peeled
- 8 ounces vegan cream cheese
- 1/4 cup vanilla soy-based yogurt
- 1 tablespoon honey
- 1-1/2 teaspoons cinnamon
- 1/4 cup brown sugar substitute
- 1/3 cup water
- 2 tablespoons cornstarch
- 2 tablespoons unsalted margarine

INSTRUCTIONS:

1. Set the Neufchatel cheese out on the counter to come to room temperature for at least 8 hours.
2. Cook up the cinnamon sauce by combining the brown sugar, water, butter, cornstarch, and a 1/2 teaspoon cinnamon over medium heat.
3. Constantly stirring, cook the mixture until the butter has melted and it begins to thicken.
4. Remove from heat and transfer to a mixing bowl; refrigerate until ready to serve.
5. Whip the cheese, using an electric mixer, in a large mixing bowl until it is a smooth, creamy texture.
6. Place the mixing bowl under the fruit chute.
7. Push frozen bananas through the fruit chute.
8. Add yogurt, honey and 1 teaspoon cinnamon to the mixing bowl.
9. Mix together until smooth and serve.

Nutritional Info: Calories: 494, Sodium: 221mg, Dietary Fiber: 7.8g, Total Fat: 16.4g, Total Carbs: 83.0g, Protein: 8.9g.

Stracciatella Ice Cream

Stracciatella is a unique blend of ice cream and olive oil that packs one savory, yet sweet, Italian style punch full of flavor. If you are looking for the ultimate antioxidant packed soft-serve, whip up a bowl of olive oil stracciatella ice cream. Neither your soul nor your skin will be disappointed!

YIELD: 3-5 SERVINGS | PREP TIME: 1 HOUR 5 MINUTES | COOK TIME: 5 MINUTES

INGREDIENTS:

- 12 frozen bananas, peeled
- 1/2 cup Greek vanilla soy-based yogurt
- 2 teaspoons cocoa powder
- 1/4 cup extra virgin olive oil (the higher the quality, the better the taste)
- 1/4 cup 85% dark cacao bar, chopped

INSTRUCTIONS:

1. Whip the cocoa powder into the yogurt until smooth.
2. Place in the refrigerator to set for 1 hour.
3. Place the mixing bowl under the fruit chute and push frozen bananas through the fruit chute.
4. Add chocolate yogurt and olive oil to the mixing bowl.
5. Mix together until smooth.
6. Fold in dark chocolate chunks.
7. Spoon into individual bowls, and freeze leftovers in an airtight container.

Nutritional Info: Calories: 375, Sodium: 15mg, Dietary Fiber: 8.8g, Total Fat: 12.3g, Total Carbs: 68.8g, Protein: 7.3g.

Berry Ice Cream with Goat Cheese

Creamy goat cheese makes for one seriously decadent, lush dessert. Mixed with the tart of berries, you'll fall in love with this soft-serve. Enjoy berry goat cheese sherbet on its own, with delicious gluten-free vanilla wafers, or dolloped into your favorite party punch!

YIELD: 3-5 SERVINGS | PREP TIME: 5 MINUTES | COOK TIME: 5 MINUTES

INGREDIENTS:

- 2 cups frozen strawberries, stemmed
- 1 cup frozen blueberries, stemmed
- 1 cup raspberries, fresh or frozen (my adjustment instead of a pound of blueberries)
- 1 teaspoon brown sugar substitute
- 2 tablespoons brandy, frozen
- 2 teaspoons lemon juice, frozen
- 4 ounces vegan goat cheese

INSTRUCTIONS:

1. Set the vegan goat cheese out and let it come to room temperature.
2. Place the mixing bowl under the fruit chute and push the frozen strawberries, blueberries and raspberries through the chute.
3. Add brown sugar, brandy, lemon juice and goat cheese to the mixing bowl.
4. Mix together until smooth using an electric hand mixer.
5. Spoon into individual bowls.

Nutritional Info: Calories: 177, Sodium: 80mg, Dietary Fiber: 3.5g, Total Fat: 8.5g, Total Carbs: 12.9g, Protein: 7.8g.

Red Velvet Ice Cream

Whip up one genuinely sinfully sweet treat when you make red velvet ice cream. This recipe is for those with one seriously sweet tooth that loves to indulge in all things scrumptiously sweet. Serve this for birthdays or for family gatherings. Red velvet ice cream is also super-kid chef friendly for rainy day activities.

YIELD: 4 SERVINGS | PREP TIME: 1 HOUR 5 MINUTES | COOK TIME: 5 MINUTES

INGREDIENTS:

- 12 frozen bananas, peeled
- 1/2 cup vanilla soy-based yogurt
- 1 teaspoon cocoa powder
- 3 tablespoons chocolate soymilk
- 1/2 cup gluten-free shortcakes, chopped into pieces
- 1/2 cup gluten-free brownies, chopped into pieces
- 3 teaspoons rainbow sprinkles

INSTRUCTIONS:

1. Whip the cocoa powder into the yogurt until smooth.
2. Place in the refrigerator to set for 1 hour.
3. Place the mixing bowl under the fruit chute and push the bananas through the chute.
4. Add chocolate soy yogurt and chocolate milk to the mixing bowl.
5. Mix together until smooth.
6. Evenly distribute chopped shortcake and brownies into individual bowls.
7. Spoon ice cream on top of cake bites and top with rainbow sprinkles.

Nutritional Info: Calories: 414, Sodium: 56.2mg, Dietary Fiber: 9.8g, Total Fat: 5.6g, Total Carbs: 94.1g, Protein: 8.0g.

Macaroon Ice Cream Torte

Sometimes you want something just a bit more decadent when it comes to making soft-serve, and this macaroon ice cream torte is just the dessert. Perfect for brunch or parties, this torte delivers decadent, rich flavor one sinfully sweet bite at a time.

YIELD: 5-8 SERVINGS | PREP TIME: 2 HOUR 5 MINUTES | COOK TIME: 5 MINUTES

INGREDIENTS:

- 24 frozen bananas, peeled
- 1 teaspoon espresso powder
- 1 cup coconut cream, chilled
- 30 chocolate macaroon cookies, crumbled
- 1 cup Heath candy bars, coarsely chopped
- 1/2 cup hot fudge topping, warmed

INSTRUCTIONS:

1. Place the mixing bowl under the fruit chute and push the bananas through the chute.
2. Add coconut cream and espresso powder to the mixing bowl.
3. Mix together until smooth.
4. Sprinkle a third of the cookies into an ungreased 9-in. springform pan. Layer with 2 cups coffee ice cream, another third of the cookies, 2 cups chocolate ice cream and 1/2 cup toffee bits; repeat layers.
5. Freeze, covered, for two hours or until firm. Slice and serve topped with warm hot fudge.

Nutritional Info: Calories: 760.3, Sodium: 29.5mg, Dietary Fiber: 18.1g, Total Fat: 25.4g, Total Carbs: 141g, Protein: 53.5g.

Lemongrass Ginger Coconut Ice Cream

Fresh lemongrass blended with the spice of ginger will light your coconut ice cream on fire. Perfect for a warm summer day, this dessert is also delicious in a gluten-free waffle cone or served atop a scoop of coconut sticky rice.

YIELD: 3 SERVINGS | PREP TIME: 5 MINUTES | COOK TIME: 5 MINUTES

INGREDIENTS:

- 2 cups frozen coconut meat
- 2 stalks of frozen lemongrass, cut into slices
- 1 tablespoon fresh ginger, grated
- 1 cup coconut cream, chilled
- 1 tablespoon honey

INSTRUCTIONS:

1. Place a mixing bowl under the fruit chute and push the coconut and lemongrass through.
2. Add grated ginger, coconut cream and honey to the mixing bowl.
3. Blend until smooth.
4. Spoon into single servings.

Nutritional Info: Calories: 445, Sodium: 26mg, Dietary Fiber: 6.8g, Total Fat: 37.2g, Total Carbs: 30.9g, Protein: 4.6g.

Watermelon Ice Cream

Sweet juice watermelon frozen at its peak makes for some seriously juicy ice cream. Packed with dairy friendly ingredients you can't go wrong with this healthy treat. Enjoy it as a snack or alongside granary toast topped with avocado for something different on your healthy diet.

YIELD: 2-4 SERVINGS | PREP TIME: 5 MINUTES | COOK TIME: 5 MINUTES

INGREDIENTS:

- 3 cups frozen watermelon, seeded
- 1/2 cup cream of coconut, chilled
- 1 teaspoon honey

INSTRUCTIONS:

1. Place the mixing bowl under the fruit chute and push the watermelon through the chute.
2. Add coconut cream and honey to the mixing bowl.
3. Mix together until smooth.
4. Spoon into individual bowls and freeze leftovers.

Nutritional Info: Calories: 248, Sodium: 2mg, Dietary Fiber: 0.8g, Total Fat: 20.2g, Total Carbs: 16.6g, Protein: 2.8g.

Rhubarb Ice Cream

Get the most out of the health benefits of when you whip up some delicious Rhubarb ice cream. Rhubarb is packed with protein, B vitamins, Vitamin C & K, as well as calcium. You'll never know this is one healthy dessert either because it tastes like a dream!

YIELD: 2-4 SERVINGS | PREP TIME: 5 MINUTES | COOK TIME: 5 MINUTES

INGREDIENTS:

- 9 stalks of frozen Rhubarb, cut into slices
- 1/4 cup vanilla soy-based yogurt
- 1/4 cup cream of coconut, chilled
- 1 teaspoon honey

INSTRUCTIONS:

1. Place a mixing bowl under the fruit chute and push the rhubarb through.
2. Add yogurt, cream of coconut and honey to the mixing bowl, and blend until smooth.
3. Spoon into individual bowl or ice cream cones.
4. Freeze leftover soft-serve in an airtight container.

Nutritional Info: Calories: 139, Sodium: 9mg, Dietary Fiber: 2.2g, Total Fat: 10.6g, Total Carbs: 9.1g, Protein: 3.5g.

Peanut Butter and Jelly Ice Cream

Turn a timeless classic into a succulently sweet soft-serve in just minutes. As simple as the combination itself, this is one easy soft serve recipe to whip up. Enjoy it with crushed animal crackers or pretzels on top for a devilishly decadent dessert.

YIELD: 3-5 SERVINGS | PREP TIME: 1 HOUR 5 MINUTES | COOK TIME: 5 MINUTES

INGREDIENTS:

- 10 frozen bananas, peeled
- 1/2 cup vanilla soy-based yogurt
- 3 tablespoons natural peanut butter, no sugar added
- 1/4 cup strawberry or red currant preserves

INSTRUCTIONS:

1. Place the mixing bowl under the fruit chute and push the bananas through the chute.
2. Add yogurt and peanut butter to the mixing bowl.
3. Mix together until smooth.
4. Fold preserves into the ice cream.
5. Scoop into individual bowls and top with your favorite treat.

Nutritional Info: Calories: 291, Sodium: 6mg, Dietary Fiber: 7.1g, Total Fat: 6.2g, Total Carbs: 58.7g, Protein: 6.6g.

Amaretto-Coffee Ice Cream

Turn this gorgeous after dinner drink into a soft-serve that is out of this world. Decadent, smooth and seriously full of coffee—you'll want to wind down every dinner party with something this rich! Try serving it with gluten-free biscotti for an even more posh dessert.

YIELD: 1 SERVINGS | PREP TIME: 5 MINUTES | COOK TIME: 15 MINUTES

INGREDIENTS:

- 3 frozen bananas, peeled
- 1/2 cup vanilla soy-based yogurt
- 1/2 teaspoon espresso powder
- 2 ounces amaretto
- 1/2 cup fresh brewed coffee
- 1/3 cup ice
- 3 creme de pirouline cookies, crushed

INSTRUCTIONS:

1. Whip the espresso powder into the yogurt until smooth and set aside.
2. Brew fresh coffee and set aside to ice.
3. Place a large mixing bowl under the fruit chute and push the bananas through.
4. Fold the espresso yogurt into the soft-serve until well-blended.
5. Add a few cubes of ice to a small rocks style glass and add coffee.
6. Top with creme de pirouline cookies and enjoy!

Nutritional Info: Calories: 806, Sodium: 4530mg, Dietary Fiber: 9.2g, Total Fat: 13.5g, Total Carbs: 113g, Protein: 37.1g.

Banana-Coconut Ice Cream

There's something so very sinful about the blend of sweet creamy coconut and sweet creamy bananas. When it comes to whipping up easy dairy free ice cream, this banana-coconut recipe will blow your mind. Serve it in a gluten-free waffle cone or covered in desiccated coconut for an even more sinfully sweet treat.

YIELD: 2-4 SERVINGS | PREP TIME: 5 MINUTES | COOK TIME: 5 MINUTES

INGREDIENTS:

- 8 frozen bananas, peeled
- 1/2 cup frozen coconut meat
- 1/2 cup coconut cream, chilled
- 1 teaspoon honey

INSTRUCTIONS:

1. Place a large mixing bowl under the fruit chute and push the bananas and coconut meat through the chute.
2. Fold the coconut cream and honey into the soft-serve until well-blended.
3. Spoon into individual bowls and freeze any leftover soft-serve in an airtight container.

Nutritional Info: Calories: 320, Sodium: 9mg, Dietary Fiber: 7.7g, Total Fat: 11.3g, Total Carbs: 58.5g, Protein: 3.6g.

Lemon Drop Sorbet

Enjoy one seriously rich, tart dessert when you whip up Lemon Drop Sorbet. Just like the shot, this dessert is spiked with vodka. Simply blend with fresh Meyer lemons for the most tantalizing treat you've ever had!

YIELD: 2 SERVINGS | PREP TIME: 5 MINUTES | COOK TIME: 5 MINUTES

INGREDIENTS:

- 4 frozen bananas, peeled
- 4 tablespoons fresh lemon juice, frozen
- 3 tablespoons lemon zest
- 1 teaspoon honey
- 1 tablespoon vodka
- 1/2 teaspoon pink Himalayan salt

INSTRUCTIONS:

1. Place a large mixing bowl under the fruit chute.
2. Push the frozen bananas through the chute.
3. Add frozen lemon juice, zest, honey, vodka and salt to mixing bowl.
4. Mix until well-blended.
5. Spoon into individual bowls.
6. Freeze leftovers in an airtight container.

Nutritional Info: Calories: 250, Sodium: 590mg, Dietary Fiber: 6.8g, Total Fat: 1.1g, Total Carbs: 59.3g, Protein: 3.0g.

Chocolate Coconut Ice Cream Sandwiches

If you've been looking for the perfect way to enjoy vegan chocolate, this is the best frozen dessert that is so easy to make.

YIELD: 4 SERVINGS | PREP TIME: 5 MINUTES | COOK TIME: 15 MINUTES

INGREDIENTS:

- 2 cups frozen coconut chunks (meat)
- 1 cup coconut cream, chilled
- 2 tablespoons sugar substitute
- 1 teaspoon pure vanilla extract
- 6 vegan chocolate cookies

INSTRUCTIONS:

1. Place a mixing bowl under the fruit chute.
2. Push the coconut meat through.
3. Add the coconut cream, sugar and vanilla extract.
4. Mix until well-blended.
5. Spoon 1 tablespoon onto a cookie and shape it to be flat on top using the spoon.
6. Top with a second cookie.
7. Repeat until all ice cream sandwiches are made.
8. Freeze leftover soft-serve in an airtight container.

Nutritional Info: Calories: 494, Sodium: 261mg, Dietary Fiber: 6.3g, Total Fat: 33.6g, Total Carbs: 45.9g, Protein: 5.5g.

Chocolate Hazelnut Ice Cream

One very special soft-serve adapted from one of Ginevra Iverson's world renowned recipe collection, a chef and former owner of Calliope in New York. You'll want to make extra to enjoy this decadent, mouth-watering ice cream all week long because this stuff blows Nutella out of the water!

YIELD: 2-4 SERVINGS | PREP TIME: 5 MINUTES | COOK TIME: 5 MINUTES

INGREDIENTS:

- 12 frozen bananas, peeled
- 1/4 cup gianduja chocolate paste
- 1/2 cup vanilla soy-based yogurt
- 3 tablespoons sugar substitute
- 1/2 cup coconut cream, chilled
- 1/4 cup hazelnuts

INSTRUCTIONS:

1. Place a mixing bowl under the fruit chute and push the bananas through.
2. Add gianduja paste, yogurt, sugar and coconut cream; mix until smooth.
3. Fold in hazelnuts.
4. Scoop into individual bowls and freeze leftovers in an airtight container.

Nutritional Info: Calories: 625.25, Sodium: 27mg, Dietary Fiber: 10.3g, Total Fat: 23.9g, Total Carbs: 105.2g, Protein: 13.1g.

Sweet Corn Ice Cream

Combine the cream of the south with sweet corn to make one sincerely delicious old-fashioned style dessert. Serve it with gluten-free waffles or on top of sweet buttered cornbread for a different kind of dessert that you might just fall in love with!

YIELD: 2-4 SERVINGS | PREP TIME: 5 MINUTES | COOK TIME: 5 MINUTES

INGREDIENTS:

- 2 bags frozen corn
- 1/2 cup kefir, plain, frozen into cubes
- 1 teaspoon vanilla flavor almond milk, frozen into cubes

INSTRUCTIONS:

1. Place a large mixing bowl under the fruit chute and push the bananas and coconut meat through the chute.
2. Fold the kefir and almond milk into the soft-serve until well-blended.
3. Spoon into individual bowls and freeze any leftover soft-serve in an airtight container.

Nutritional Info: Calories: 142.75, Sodium: 19.75mg, Dietary Fiber: 3.6g, Total Fat: 1.35g, Total Carbs: 32.2g, Protein: 142.8g.

Cookies and Ice Cream

Creamy vanilla soft-serve blended with chunks of chocolate crème filled cookies is just out of this world—especially when it is super-healthy and packed full of potassium and antioxidants. This dairy free dessert is best served simply on its own.

YIELD: 4-6 SERVINGS | PREP TIME: 5 MINUTES | COOK TIME: 5 MINUTES

INGREDIENTS:

- 16 frozen bananas, peeled
- 1 cup coconut cream, chilled
- 1 cup vegan chocolate crème filled cookies, crumbled

INSTRUCTIONS:

1. Place a mixing bowl under the fruit chute and push the bananas through.
2. Add coconut cream to the mixing bowl and blend until smooth.
3. Fold in cookie crumbles.
4. Serve in individual bowls and freeze leftover soft-serve in an airtight container.

Nutritional Info: Calories: 453, Sodium: 117mg, Dietary Fiber: 9.7g, Total Fat: 13.2g, Total Carbs: 87.6g, Protein: 5.6g.

Fruity Frozen Yogurt

Fresh frozen fruit is absolutely refreshing when you turn it into a delicious frozen yogurt. Enjoy this succulently sweet treat for dessert, as an afternoon snack or alongside gluten-free biscotti for a decadent healthy dessert.

YIELD: 5 SERVINGS | PREP TIME: 5 MINUTES | COOK TIME: 5 MINUTES

INGREDIENTS:

- 3 frozen bananas, peeled
- 3 cups frozen mixed fruit
- 1/2 cup vanilla soy-based yogurt
- 1 tablespoon fresh lemon juice

INSTRUCTIONS:

1. Place a large mixing bowl under the fruit chute.
2. Push frozen bananas through the chute followed by the frozen mixed fruits.
3. Add yogurt and lemon juice to mixing bowl.
4. Mix until smooth.
5. Spoon into individual bowls.
6. Freeze leftovers in an airtight container.

Nutritional Info: Calories: 117, Sodium: 18mg, Dietary Fiber: 3.6g, Total Fat: 0.6g, Total Carbs: 27.6g, Protein: 2.2g.

CHAPTER 8
Bonus

Pantry: What to Have On Hand for These Desserts

When it comes to stocking your pantry for the ultimate fruit based soft-serve, there are a lot of supplies and items you should always have on hand. From frozen fruit to nuts, non-dairy and other diet-friendly topping options, this comprehensive list of ingredients can help you keep the healthy soft-serve flowing out of your kitchen with great ease.

Ripe Bananas

Most of the recipes call for a base of bananas. Ripe frozen bananas are always the best thing to constantly keep in your freezer for endless fun! Simply pick up a bunch of overripe bananas at your local grocer, peel, and place in a freezer safe bag. You might want to write the date on the bag in permanent marker, so you remember when you froze them. If you keep ripe frozen bananas on hand, you can create the most basic of the fruit based frozen soft-serve.

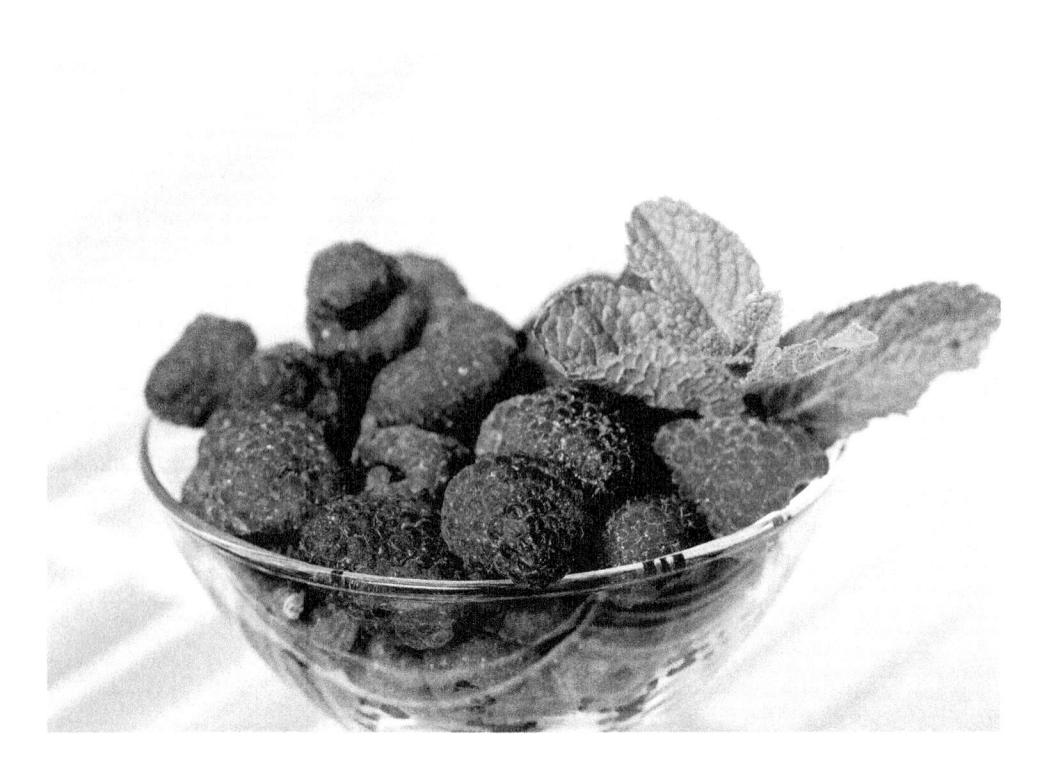

Frozen Fruits

If you love your fruit based soft-serve you might want to keep bags of fresh frozen fruit on hand for the super-delicious specialty recipes. Frozen bags of fruit are easily accessible from your local grocer's freezer. You can even order specialty frozen fruits online for endless frozen treat fun. Frozen fruits to consider in bagged options are:

- Strawberries
- Blueberries
- Raspberries
- Mixed berries
- Mango
- Cassis
- Mulberries
- Apricots
- Rhubarb
- Dark Cherries
- Pineapple
- Papaya
- Nuts

Add an explosion of savory or salty taste to your favorite fruit based soft-serve by topping it with delicious, healthy, and nutritious nuts. Nuts, especially tree nuts, are absolutely decadent and pack a healthy punch. A great source of energy, nuts are also packed with essential amino acids; as well as Vitamin E, B2 and a whole lot of tummy filling fiber. Topping your ice cream with nuts will help you feel fuller longer and keep the snacking to a minimum.

Scrumptious nuts that can be chopped up for toppings include:

- Almonds
- Brazil Nuts
- Cacao
- Cashews
- Chestnuts
- Coconut
- Hazelnuts
- Macadamia
- Peanuts
- Pistachios
- Walnuts
- Betel Nuts
- Kola Nuts
- Pecans
- Pine Nut

Types of Non-Dairy/Paleo Diet Friendly Toppings

The best part about whipping up fruit based soft-serve is that you can also top it just like you would in a dairy bar, ice cream parlor, or froyo-style shop. We love the endless toppings just as much as you do! When exploring soft-serve, we learned you just have to think outside the box. Luckily for you, we compiled some of the most yummy, tantalizing treats to top your soft-serve with! If you're wild about toppings, here are our favorite dairy-free/paleo diet friendly options:

- Fresh Berries
- Chopped Stone Fruit like Nectarines, Peaches, Cherries, Apricots and Dates
- Diced Banana
- Minced Herbs like Mint, Lemongrass, Basil, Rosemary and Thyme
- Crushed Potato Chips, Pretzels or Popcorn (these are gluten-free options too!)
- Mango Chutney
- Graham Crackers (these come in a gluten-free option too!)
- Tropical Powder
- Freeze-Dried Fruit
- Raisins
- Let's Do Organic Sprinkelz that comes in Confetti, Chocolate or Coconut
- Dandies Vegan Marshmallows
- Crushed up YumEarth Candies like Peppermint, Butterscotch & Root Beer
- Sultry Crystallized Ginger
- Dairy-Free Chocolate Chips that come in several versions: Mini, Chunks or Organic Dark
- Juicy Mandarin Oranges
- Flaked or Shredded Coconut
- Chopped Tropical Fruit like Papaya, Pineapple, Passion fruit, and more
- So Delicious CocoWhip
- Girl Scout Cookies: Thin Mints
- Organic Candy Factory Jelly Beans

- Surf Sweets Gummy Bears and Worms
- Yummy Chocolate-Covered Chia or Hemp Seeds
- Lucy's Crunchy Cookies (these guys come in loads of flavors!)
- Justin's Dark Chocolate Peanut Butter Cups (simply to die for!)
- NoNo's (The Dairy Free Sixlet for you 80's kids)
- Cookie Dough
- Chopped Go Max Go Candy Bars (Oh yes, they are just like Snickers, Butterfingers and Milky Way - just to mention a few)
- Trader Joe's Cookie Butter
- Mylk Chocolate Frosting (because no one needs cake)
- Chocolate Covered Dates
- Navitas Naturals Coconut Chips
- I.M. Healthy Soy Nut Granola
- Earth Balance P.B. Pops
- Chocolate Chunk Granola
- Crumbled Cow Pie Cookies
- Hail Merry Macaroons
- Cacao Nibs
- Goji Berries
- Enjoy Life Soft Baked Cookies
- Granola
- Glutino Wafer Bites (these melt in your mouth!)
- Rhubarb Compote or Jam
- Maple Pecan Pralines
- Rice Mallow
- Rice Crispy Treats with Rice Mallow
- Pie Crust Crumbles

Gluten-Free Toppings

Whether you have Celiac Disease, are gluten intolerant, suffer from Candida overgrowth, or just want a healthier lifestyle without any wheat - we've got some super-delicious ideas for topping your soft-serve.

While most of the options above are gluten-free, we wanted to go the extra mile and give you gluten-free soft-serve lovers something to really savor!

- Chocolate or Honey Nut Cheerio's
- Pop Rocks

- Plain M&M's
- Fruit by The Foot
- Sriracha
- Kool Aid (Yep, just sprinkle your favorite flavor on there!)
- Marshmallow Fluff
- Espresso Ground Coffee
- Gourmet Popcorn (Think: Kettle, Caramel, Toffee, Chocolate Covered)
- Fruit Snacks
- French Fries (If you dip French fries in your chocolate frosty you know what we're talking about!)
- Peppermint Patties
- Chocolate Covered Raisins
- Haribo Gummies (This includes Star Mix & Cola Bottles)
- Fruity Pebbles
- Apple Cider (If it's alcoholic you can make drunken ice cream floats—it's delicious in cool winter months)

Natural Ingredients to Turn your Soft-Serve Sorbet into a Decadent Dessert

When it comes to whipping up your fruit based soft-serve with "out of this world" taste that is a little more on the natural side, it's just as easy as sprinkling on the toppings above. You might be thinking, mint, vanilla, essence of lavender, or rose oil. Of course if you want something a little more adventurous, you can totally go wild and turn your favorite fruit-filled soft-serve into Birthday Cake, Bubble Gum, Cotton Candy, or Black Walnut!

Natural Flavored Oils

Bakers and candy makers are no strangers to oils that infuse their confectionary treats with a plethora of different flavors that you may not be able to create with just fruit and natural additives. These oils can often be found with zero alcohol, making these flavors super paleo friendly and overall great for the healthy lifestyle that includes no sugar. Fabulous natural flavors include:

- Apple
- Bubble Gum
- Cherry
- Cotton Candy
- Grape
- Marshmallow
- Peanut Butter
- Root Beer
- Strawberry
- Tutti-Fruitti

- Almond
- Amaretto
- Anise
- Apricot
- Banana Cream
- Bavarian Cream
- Black Cherry
- Blackberry
- Black Walnut
- Blueberry
- Bourbon
- Brandy
- Butter
- Butter Rum
- Buttered Popcorn
- Butterscotch
- Caramel
- Champagne/Sparkling Wine
- Cheesecake
- Cherry Chocolate
- Chocolate Hazelnut
- Cinnamon

KITCHEN UNIT CONVERSION

1 teaspoon	=	1/3 tbsp	=	4.9 ml
1 dessertspoon	=	2 tsp	=	9.9 ml
1 tablespoon	=	1.5 dstsp / 3 tsp	=	14.8 ml
1 fuid ounce	=	2 tbsp / 6 tsp	=	29.6 ml
1 cup	=	16 tbsp / 48 tsp	=	236.6 ml
1 quart	=	4 cup	=	946 ml
1 gal	=	4 quart / 16 cup	=	3.79 l
1 ounce	=	2 tbsp	=	28.4 g
1 pounds	=	16 oz	=	453.6 g